Living with

ORAL ALLERGY SYNDROME

A gluten and meat-free cookbook for wheat, soy, nut,

fresh fruit and vegetable allergies

Living with

ORAL ALLERGY SYNDROME

A gluten and meat-free cookbook for wheat, soy, nut,

fresh fruit and vegetable allergies

❧ **Danielle S. LeBlanc** ☙

With foreword by
Rod LeBlanc, DTCM

La Venta West Publishers

Vancouver, Canada

La Venta West Publishers
Vancouver, Canada
www.laventawestpublishers.blogspot.com

Disclaimers: *This book is intended as an informational guide. The remedies and techniques described herein are for educational purposes only, and not meant as a substitute for professional medical care or treatment. Please read the suggested contents of each recipe carefully and determine whether or not they may create a problem for you. All recipes are used at the risk of the consumer.*

We are not responsible for any hazards, loss or damage that may occur as a result of any recipe use or use of information provided herein. In the event of any doubt, please contact your medical advisor prior to use.

Photo credits: Danielle LeBlanc
Cover design: idrewdesign @fiverr.com
Cover photos: *Tenerumi Noodle Soup* page 96
                   Chickpea Flatbread page 76
Back cover: *Chocolate Beet Muffins and Cupcakes* page 78
                   Thai Noodle Salad page 88
                   Spiced Chocolate Applesauce Cake page 124
                   Chilled Pear Soup page 123

ISBN 978-0-9920802-0-4

Acknowledgements:

In gratitude to my husband, Alexander, for his constant support and his willingness to implement the "try one new food thing per day" rule, even when it looked sketchy. This book could never have happened without him.

To both my parents for teaching me to cook, each in their own unique way. To mum, for buying me my first cookbook for my 7th birthday, and to dad, for teaching me to use chopsticks and beginning to unravel the allergy mystery.

Special thanks to Lindsay, Randy and Michael for their enthusiasm for this project, and ready willingness to work around my allergy list at family dinners.

❧ CONTENTS ❦

Foreword by
Dr. Rod LeBlanc
Doctor of Traditional Chinese Medicine

Having allergies can be an isolating experience. Over the years I have seen multiple patients with hay fever and related food allergies who live in fear of food and allergic reactions. Social events and outdoor activities can be stress inducing, and can cause embarrassment. Some feel like it's easier to just stay home than battle potentially dangerous restaurant menus, buffets and potlucks, explaining their allergies to everyone along the way.

There is also a psychology of guilt and blaming that goes along with allergies, particularly in the case of little-understood fresh fruit and vegetable allergies. Allergy sufferers are told (or themselves believe) that they have done something to cause their allergies; genes, poor immunity, toxic self, over-exertion, diet, etc. Some people are even told that their legitimate allergies are psychosomatic and self-induced; they're "imagined", "made up to get attention" or "an excuse to complain", or they are "just being picky and difficult".

At the same time, many live in total denial or are unaware that food allergies could be a culprit in their health problems. Food allergies can lead to eczema, hives, abdominal pain, nausea, asthmatic symptoms, feelings of lethargy, and more. Furthermore, foods that cause allergic reactions also cause inflammation. Inflammation can lead to arthritis, joint and muscle pain, fibromyalgia, depression, gut acidity, etc. Patients are typically prescribed a host of anti-inflammatories, anti-depressants and other medications to treat symptoms, but the underlying cause too often goes undiagnosed and problems worsen. Allergies are autoimmune conditions that tie into other autoimmune conditions and, if left untreated, this can become a degenerative cycle.

Researchers are just starting to track how allergies are created in our environment while the human race is becoming more prone to wide-spread autoimmune diseases, connective tissue disorders and allergies. Through Danielle's careful research of oral allergy syndrome, she presents a coherent explanation of how our immune systems have become inexplicably compromised in recent years as a result of a combination of chemicals, our environment, pollutants in our air and our damaged food system.

This oral allergy syndrome book is remarkable in its scope, providing not only a wealth of information on food allergies, but also a means for people to begin to cope with some of their debilitating physical and mental repercussions. Our immune systems have become weaker with each decade and allergies are now seen in epidemic proportions in every clinic around the globe. The research presented in Danielle's book provides a useful link to our understanding of allergies, their underlying causes and the use of safe food as a source of nutrition. The healthy and enticing dishes offer a means of incorporating healthy foods into an oral allergy syndrome diet.

Most importantly, Danielle's book provides assistance for those who wish to take power over their diet and work towards healing some of the ailments associated with oral allergy syndrome.

Rod LeBlanc, DTCM

Founder of the Lifelong Health Clinic and the Society for Acupoint Injection Therapy (SAIT)

September 2013, White Rock, BC

✤ Introduction ✤

Have you ever found yourself scanning the pollen counts for the next week, dreading the onset of allergy season? If so, it's quite possible you've also experienced oral allergy syndrome (OAS, also known as food-pollen allergy), a type of food allergy associated with seasonal allergies and hay fever. OAS results from a cross-reaction between pollens such as birch, ragweed, mugwort, grass and latex and a wide variety of fresh fruits, vegetables, nuts, soy and wheat. If you or your child has ever inexplicably experienced tingling, discomfort, itchiness, hives or stomach upset after eating certain foods, for example an apple, peach or almonds, you may have OAS. Some people also experience similar reactions to meat and milk, although these are not necessarily related to hay fever.

This book not only provides insight into OAS, it also has tons of tips, tricks and recipes to help you take control of your diet and health. Being informed and understanding your allergies can enable you to put fruits and vegetables back into your meals while working towards healing your body and eating a balanced diet.

✤ The leading cause of food allergies and sensitivities ✤

Although little known at present, *oral allergy syndrome is the leading cause of food allergies* amongst children and adults,[1] and studies suggest that up to 55-70% of food allergies are related to OAS.[2] While it is difficult to determine the exact percentage of people with it (as explained below), the percentage of people with OAS is estimated to be very high in some countries. For example, in 2004 a German study found a reported rate of 3.7% percent of people had food allergies, with OAS as the main cause.[3] In a small study of Mexican adults with hay fever, 13% of the participants were found to suffer from OAS.[4] Other studies that pertain to hay fever suggest that anywhere between 30-90% of people with hay fever also have OAS.[5]

If one begins to do the math, it becomes apparent that *there are likely tens of millions of people around the world suffering from oral allergy syndrome*. For example, the FDA estimates that 35 million people in the US suffer from hay fever.[6] If 30 – 90% of these people are also afflicted with OAS than it is possible that anywhere between 10.5 and 31.5 million people in the US alone are suffering from allergies related to wheat, soy, apples, peaches, nuts and other related foods.

The percentage of people with oral allergy syndrome is difficult to determine for several reasons. First, **the term oral allergy syndrome (OAS) has only been in use since 1987,** when it was first proposed by scientists to describe the reactions some people experienced around the mouth area after eating particular foods.[7] Second, most of the research on OAS is inaccessible without pricey subscriptions to scientific journals.

Thankfully, over the course of my graduate studies I was able to access and rigorously search various scientific journals in order to better understand the allergies that I myself was struggling with. I am lucky to be able to continue my research today, and since January of 2011 I have shared several articles on OAS and numerous recipes on my blog, www.poorandglutenfree.blogspot.com. Some of the most pertinent information I have found (and some of the most delicious recipes I have created) are shared right here in this book.

Finally, **OAS often goes unreported or undiagnosed** by doctors and patients because the symptoms people experience are usually mild,[8] rather than the severe, anaphylactic response of only a small percentage of sufferers. Sometimes doctors themselves are unfamiliar with OAS, as the information from scientific journals doesn't always trickle down to busy family doctors and allergists.

Because of this lack of awareness, oral allergy syndrome can be an extremely frustrating condition. Going without diagnosis can cause all kinds of health problems such as chronic fatigue, hives, upset stomach, migraines, malnutrition and diarrhea. I have heard from numerous people through my blog who have been diagnosed with chronic issues such as irritable bowel syndrome (IBS), fatigue, depression and fibromyalgia, only to find that they may actually have been symptoms of OAS.

Even with a diagnosis, it can be hard to figure out what to eat when you feel as if you are *allergic to everything.* It's difficult enough to eat all the daily recommended fruits and vegetables, but when suddenly the options become drastically limited it can be all the more disheartening. The **good news** is that not only are there fruits and vegetables *not* commonly associated with OAS, but studies have shown that peeling, cooking, boiling and canning certain fruits and vegetables can denature the allergen proteins, making them safer for many people with OAS to eat. This is explained in Chapter 2, and many of the recipes in this book make use of processed fruits and veggies, incorporating them into breakfasts, baked goods, soups, salads, snacks, dinners and delicious desserts.

Sadly, most of us with OAS have heard at some point from family and/or doctors that "It's all in your head", "You're just looking for an excuse to avoid eating vegetables", or "You're just trying to get attention". These accusations can lead to feelings of depression, frustration, paranoia, guilt, and shame. My own story is a prime example of the difficulties involved in diagnosing OAS.

❧ My Story ☙

I suffered from oral allergy syndrome unknowingly for at least 8 years. Symptoms began to manifest around my 20th birthday, when I suddenly developed hay fever despite not having any previous allergies. Shortly afterwards I began to notice that my mouth and throat felt itchy and tight after eating almonds. Within a few years I developed an inexplicable aversion to most fresh fruits and vegetables. They made me *uncomfortable*, and I couldn't explain why.

It culminated one year when the pollen counts were exceptionally high. I experienced chronic exhaustion and brain fog, and I developed painful hives all over my back. Each night I coughed so much I could hardly sleep and my stomach and throat ached the next day. I saw two different doctors who each gave me inhalers for asthma, nose sprays for my allergies and offered acne medication for the hives. However, testing showed I didn't have asthma, the inhalers didn't help, the sprays painfully dried out my nostrils and I refused the acne medication.

Furthermore, I somehow contracted pink eye *in both eyes*, and got a sinus infection that was so bad it plugged my left ear. My doctor prescribed antibiotics, but I refused them as I suspected that they would only further damage my system (it turns out I was right, as I explain in Chapter 1). Instead, I healed my own sinus infection with regular sinus rinses, facial steaming, and warm oil dripped into my ear. ***All in all, though, I was a total mess!*** I didn't even want to visit friends because I was so embarrassed by my appearance and constant coughing, sneezing, sniffling and miserable mood. I felt like I was a burden to be around.

My family doctor tested me for anaemia and hypothyroidism with negative results. My father, Rod LeBlanc, a doctor of Traditional Chinese Medicine, suggested I might have an issue with gluten and food intolerance, so I asked my family doctor to test me for celiac disease. Negative results again, although I have since discovered my father was right and I am gluten intolerant. The doctor suggested that I might be depressed. I refused to believe it. I knew there had to be some reason *all* of these problems were happening at once.

I pressed to see an allergist and, after a scratch test that left my arm with giant welts and a brutal elimination diet, I found that I was gluten intolerant and allergic to almost everything. Unsatisfied with the allergist's suggested treatment of immunization shots that "may or may not help," I went on to do my own research.

I was incredibly disappointed and frustrated that throughout all of this I had to ask and press for information and assistance. *Had I left it to regular doctors, I would have been on steroidal anti-histamines, asthma inhalers, penicillin, anti-depressants and acne medication all at the same time!* And in the end, all those drugs still wouldn't have solved my problems.

After several years of coping with OAS I began Poor and Gluten Free .blogspot.com in order to chronicle some of my research and allergy adventures and to share recipes. The comments I've received from readers strongly indicated that people need more information about OAS. I decided to bring all my research and some of my best recipes together into this book in the hope that it might help prevent other people from having to suffer like me, as well as foster awareness of OAS and encourage more research.

Ultimately, there are several key things I've learned that I hope to impart to those of you learning to live with oral allergy syndrome.

* *You are not imagining it.* Food allergies are real, and if you think you are allergic to something, get tested and find out.

* *Trust and listen to your body.* If something feels *off*, it probably is.

* *It's not your fault.* Allergies are caused by a wide variety of factors, most of which are well beyond your control.

* *You are not alone.* Millions of other people suffer from food allergies, and not just to peanuts or dairy.

* *You can be healthy and happy, even with multiple food allergies.* Take this as an opportunity to learn more about your health and well-being. Allergies are a good reason to pay attention to what's in your food and your environment, and to share your experiences with others to raise awareness.

* *Maintain a positive attitude and be thankful when you learn what your allergies are.* It sounds crazy, right? Nobody rejoices when they hear they're allergic to almost everything. But once you know what you are

reactive to, you can begin to control the allergens in your environment and work towards achieving your optimal health, instead of continuing to suffer from mysterious ailments.

Since I myself am allergic to most OAS related foods, I know how difficult it can be to cook and dine out with so many food allergies. My own frustration has prompted years of experimentation and what I've found has enabled me to incorporate many of the offending foods back in to my diet. Here I've shared my research and recipes in the hopes that others might benefit and learn to live better with oral allergy syndrome.

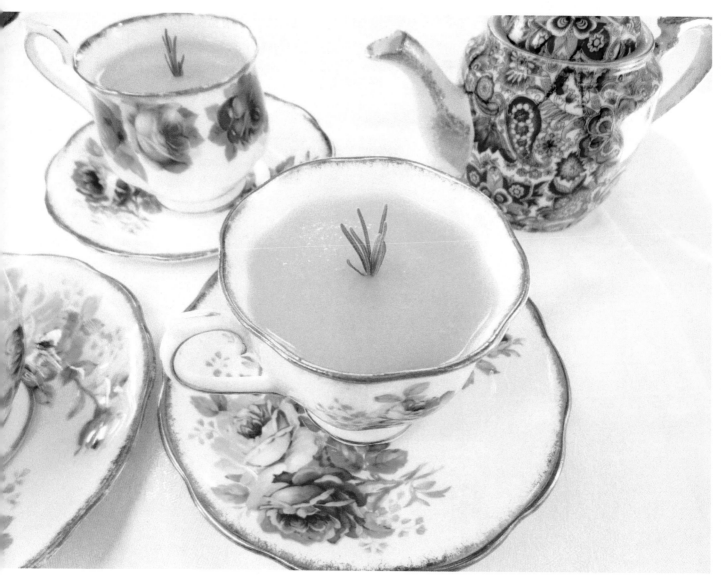

Chilled Pear Soup

❧ Chapter 1 ❧

Understanding Oral Allergy Syndrome

(a.k.a. Pollen-Food Allergy)

❧ What is oral allergy syndrome? ❧

OAS is the term used to describe the allergic reaction some people have to foods that are related to birch, grass, mugwort, cypress or ragweed pollen, as well as latex (also known as latex-fruit syndrome).[9] Some of the foods people most commonly react to include apples, hazelnuts, wheat, almonds, kiwi, carrots, celery, peaches, cherries, strawberries and soy (See Table 1 for a more complete list).

Oral allergy syndrome is unlike other food allergies because unlike peanut allergies for example, the severity of the symptoms can wax and wane with the season. OAS does not begin on its own, but is triggered by allergies to certain pollens.

For those who suffer from OAS, the problems probably began with the typical hay fever symptoms: itchy eyes and stuffy noses during allergy season. Likely, it then progressed to an uncomfortable itchiness or swelling of the mouth or throat after eating certain foods. This might have been imperceptible in its early stages, or maybe even just an inexplicable aversion to certain foods. While some children grow out of childhood allergies, many do not. A large number of adults can develop oral allergy syndrome after their teens[10] and these can be a lifelong problem.

❧ What are the symptoms? ❧

Foods associated with OAS can cause tingling, itchiness and swelling of the mouth, tongue and throat. Skin rashes such as hives, blisters, and painful atopic dermatitis (eczema) are also not uncommon. Some experience stomach upset and indigestion, shortness of breath and, in severe cases, anaphylactic shock. Symptoms manifest within 5 minutes to several hours after contacting food and are most often limited to the mouth and throat, although symptoms can vary depending on the severity of the allergy. Some can develop itchy rashes on areas of their skin that have come in contact with the offending food.[11]

Food most commonly associated with Oral Allergy Syndrome[12]	
Birch (includes the Alder family)	**Fruits**: apple, apricot, cherry, date, kiwi, nectarine, peach, pear, plum, prune, tomato* **Vegetables**: anise/fennel, beans, bell pepper*, carrot, celery, parsnip, pea, potato, soybean **Nuts, Seeds & Grains**: almond, caraway, buckwheat, hazelnut, lentils, peanut, sunflower, walnut, wheat **Herbs**: coriander, cumin, dill, fennel, parsley **Others**: honey (pollen)
Grass	**Fruits**: kiwi, melon, orange, tomato*, watermelon
Mugwort	**Fruits**: apple, melons (i.e. cantaloupe, honeydew, watermelon) **Vegetables**: carrot, celery
Ragweed	**Fruits**: banana, melons (i.e. cantaloupe, honeydew, watermelon) **Vegetables**: cucumber*, zucchini* **Others**: honey
Cypress[13] (includes Japanese Cedar)	**Fruits**: peach **Vegetables**: lettuce, mustard **Nuts**: hazelnut
Latex	**Fruits**: banana, peach, kiwi **Vegetables**: avocado, bell pepper*, potato, tomato* **Nuts**: chestnut
Meats and Milk	Pork, beef, chicken, turkey, milk**
* These foods are botanically classified as fruits, but often considered to be vegetables ** Not typically associated with hay fever, but can induce adverse oral and topical reactions	

Table 1 OAS Chart

The severity of the symptoms can also wax and wane along with hay fever season, with symptoms usually being at their worst during hay fever season in the spring and summer. However, although allergy season is usually short, often symptoms of OAS can remain throughout the year. So while it may be winter and pollens outside are inactive, one can still experience swelling or discomfort after eating an apple or piece of celery, for example. The body reacts to these foods with a histamine response, similar to the way it reacts to pollen during hay fever season.

Not everyone is allergic to every food item on the list. Having an allergy to birch does not necessarily mean that you will react to every single food that is associated with birch. Some people may only react to one or two items, while others may react to 20 or more. The severity of the allergy may also depend on the level of pollens in the fruit itself.

❧ What types of foods are associated with OAS? ❧

A wide variety of foods are associated with OAS. Birch in particular is believed to be the pollen that causes the most OAS symptoms, with anywhere between 30-90% of people with hay fever experiencing OAS symptoms as a result of pollen allergies.[14] Furthermore, studies from Finland estimate that 10-15% of the Finnish population are affected by birch pollen allergies, most of them accompanied by OAS-related food allergies.[15] Some of the most reactive foods associated with birch include apples, cherries, peaches, carrot, celery, almonds, hazelnuts, soy and wheat.

Meats and milk can also cause hives, shortness of breath, tingling, upset stomach and even anaphylactic shock; although at present they are not connected to hay fever. Recent research has shown that meat allergies may, in fact, be caused by tick bites.[16] Furthermore, those with milk allergies (*not lactose intolerance*) are often also allergic to beef. Although meat and milk allergies are not addressed in depth in this book as their connection to hay fever is unclear, the recipes found here are meat-free and almost all offer dairy-free alternatives, such as coconut and rice milk.

❧ How does the cross-reaction work? ❧

For whatever reason (I investigate this further in this chapter), the immune system of those of us with hay fever consider pollen as an allergen, a potentially dangerous invading army of sorts. In order to destroy these invaders, **Immunoglobulin E (IgE)**, a type of antibody made by the immune system, tracks down and binds itself to the pollen cells. Let's consider this IgE as a **Special Forces Unit** of sorts. By binding to the pollen cells, this Special Forces Unit triggers massive amounts of **histamine** to be produced, which in turn helps to dilate the blood vessels and produce more white blood cells. The body wants more white blood cells (the body's own personal **Royal Guard**, of sorts) in order to fight off the supposed invading pollen. This massive and abnormal production of histamine can trigger inflammation, irritation and contraction of the smooth muscles that can in turn cause asthmatic-like responses and allergic reactions to pollen in those of us with allergies.

It's bad enough that our bodies erroneously see pollen as a foreign invader, but then, somewhere along the way, our immune systems went into further overdrive. Something happens where certain pollens *cross-react* with various foods in related families, meaning that the pollens and foods react with one another. Therefore the body recognizes those foods as being the same as the pollen it is allergic to. Now the body not only considers pollen as a foreign invader, it considers anything related to pollen as the enemy. In a way, it's as if the Special Forces has gone from sending out the Royal Guard whenever the invaders come to town, to sending out the Royal Guard to blow up the neighbours if they stop by for dinner, *just in case...*

❧ Diagnosis of OAS ❦

There are several means of diagnosing OAS which are usually used in combination by doctors. *A scratch test* is the first step to determining what pollens and foods you are allergic to. This consists of the skin being pricked and a small amount of pollen in liquid form being dropped onto the skin to determine the results. A large area of swelling usually indicates a histamine response, and therefore an allergic reaction.

The scratch test is sometimes followed by *an oral test*, in which the potentially offensive foods are consumed in order to observe the reaction. This helps to determine exactly which foods you or your child react to, and to what degree. It is important to do this in a controlled environment with a doctor, due to the small risk of anaphylactic shock.

A *Specific Allergen IgE* test (*SAIGE*) can also be done to see if you have IgE in your system to specific foods. Blood is collected and then mixed with a particular allergen to see if the IgE binds to the allergen. High levels of IgE indicate the presence of allergic reactions. This may be done in cases where anaphylactic shock is a possibility, or for small children who may find the other tests grueling.

In some cases, an *elimination diet* is recommended in order to determine which foods cause reactions. This method involves a strict diet which slowly re-incorporates foods to determine the patient's response. This particular method can be difficult to endure due to its austere nature but can be one of the most effective ways of determining all potential food allergies and their intensity, as some of the other tests may conflict with one another (i.e. a SAIGE test may produce different results than a scratch test).

You may want to *keep a food diary* to keep track of reactions to foods and various exposures. This can help pinpoint specific allergies, or products that might contain offending foods and ingredients. For example, cosmetics can contain hydrolyzed wheat proteins. If you are allergic to wheat, exposure to hydrolyzed wheat proteins may cause hives, itchiness or shortness of breath. Keeping a diary that tracks food and exposures can determine which foods and products cause reactions.

For more on hydrolyzed wheat protein in products, you can check out this article on **Poor and Gluten Free**:

http://www.poorandglutenfree.blogspot.ca/2012/09/oral-allergy-syndrome-wheat-allergies.html

For a printable PDF diary chart, go to:

http://poorandglutenfree.blogspot.com/p/oral-allergy-syndrome.html

It is always advisable to conduct these tests under the supervision of a doctor.

❧ Is there a treatment for OAS? ❦

At present the potential treatment of OAS is still in the early stages, and results of various studies have proven to be contradictory, although there is some promising research. For example, a 2012 study in Japan found that birch pollen **immunotherapy** (i.e. allergy shots) was beneficial for a teenage girl suffering from birch pollinosis and OAS,[17] but another French study indicates that, while effective for some patients, it was not necessarily effective for everyone and much more research needs to be done.[18] In my own experience with readers' comments through my blog, immunotherapy has provided mixed results with varying degrees of efficacy ranging from some benefit to none at all. A preliminary study suggests that the use of **birch pollen honey** (honey infused with particles of birch pollen) may be effective in treating birch pollen allergies; however OAS was not taken into account in the study.[19] These studies all indicate that much more research is needed before effective treatments for OAS are made available to the public.

Some people have found relief with the use of **natural remedies and/or alternative medicine**. At present, these methods lack scientific evidence to prove 100% effectiveness but this not to say that they won't be proved effective in time. For example, some people claim to have found relief through acupuncture. Other purported natural remedies found on various personal and health and wellness blogs include; ingestion of local bee pollen or honey (which may contain trace amounts of the offending pollen, and therefore it may have results similar to immunotherapy and birch pollen honey), aromatherapy, dietary changes, and herbs such as Butterbur. More scientific research needs to be done to determine the veracity of these methods and therapies, as well as the correct method of administering them. However, there are several ways to provide relief from allergy symptoms, which are outlined later in this chapter.

Other potentially promising avenues of research have to do with **probiotics and beneficial gut flora, as well as Omega 3s**. This will be explained in more detail in the below section on causes of OAS and allergies.

❧ What Causes OAS and Allergies? ❧

Although we understand *how* bodies react to certain pollens and foods they consider invaders, at present it is unclear *why* our bodies view them as invaders in the first place. Nearly all the studies referenced in this book note that allergies are on the rise in industrialized countries (most countries report a rate of allergies between 15-35%, with the worldwide average being 22%)[20], and multiple studies have been done to determine potential causes. The results indicate that a combination of both genetic and environmental factors is likely responsible for the rise of allergies.[21] For example, genetics, an increase in exposure to allergens, pollution and irritants (such as smoke, gas and chemicals), stress, infections, dietary changes and lack of exposure to beneficial bacteria have all been suggested as playing a role in allergies.[22] While hay fever has been shown to be hereditary in some cases,[23] and hay fever is a precursor for OAS, genetics is not necessarily the strongest cause of OAS.

There are some obstacles to determining what causes OAS. First off, OAS is triggered predominantly in those with pollen allergies, a.k.a. *allergic rhinitis* (AR). Since the mystery of what specifically causes AR has yet to be solved, it is difficult to understand how or why pollen allergies lead to food allergies. The other problem with studying the cause of allergies and OAS is, as mentioned in the *Introduction*, that OAS was only named, and therefore recognized, as a condition by scientists in 1987.[24] There has been little opportunity for long term studies. It is believed that OAS generally manifests itself in adult life, or late teens, although some do experience reactions in childhood.[25] Most long-term, large-scale studies on allergies have not gone beyond the teenage years, so it is difficult to determine the potential triggers of OAS in later years.

So in order to begin to understand what causes OAS, we must turn to studies on allergic rhinitis and food allergies in general. Studies of AR have indicated both potential causes or risk factors *and* potential protections against the development of allergies. The vast majority of these studies indicate that hay fever, even if it manifests after early childhood, may be determined as early as in the womb and during infancy.

For those who feel responsible for their allergies, hopefully this will provide some vindication.

The 'hygiene hypothesis' has been gaining ground in the scientific community for some time now. Essentially, the hypothesis is that children in urban areas of industrialized countries, where rates of allergies and asthma are highest, are no longer exposed to the same amounts of microbes and bacteria as those in rural and less industrialized countries. This is due, in part, to **increased use of antibiotics and vaccinations** in early life that decrease the body's ability to develop a healthy immune system.[26] Furthermore, **a lack of infections** in early childhood, like the common cold, is actually associated with *higher* rates of allergies and asthma later in life.[27] Essentially, as a result of not having been exposed to bacteria and microbes, the body's immune system becomes stunted and immature.

Put very simply and to carry the earlier analogy to the extreme, it is as if the body's Special Forces lack the necessary basic training to do their job properly. It's as if they missed the part of training camp where they learned to recognize "friendlies" (non-enemies) and don't realize it is inappropriate to assault the neighbours (a.k.a. pollen and OAS related foods) when they arrive on the doorstep.

Respiratory infections in early childhood have also been correlated with higher rates of allergies later in life.[28] Whereas children who are exposed to more bacteria and common infections in early childhood are less likely to have allergies, those with respiratory infections such as pneumonia, bronchitis or otitis appear *more* likely to have allergies and asthma. The effect of infections doesn't manifest itself immediately as allergies can appear many years later, rather than shortly after the infection.

It had previously been suggested that the administration of **antibiotics**, such as **penicillin**, used to manage respiratory infections, were the cause of allergies and asthma. More recent studies suggest that while antibiotics are not necessarily the direct cause of allergies and immune disorders, they may play an important role in causing allergies. As mentioned above, antibiotics can stunt the development of the immune system, as well as causing a variety of side effects such as loss of gut bacteria, impaired kidney function, tendonitis, inner-ear problems, diarrhea, and hearing loss. In particular, antibiotics can cause "oxidative stress that can lead to damage to DNA, proteins and lipids in human cells."[29] It is now recommended to use antibiotics sparingly to avoid antibiotic resistance and other negative side effects.[30]

A key issue related to antibiotic use is the decrease in **beneficial gut bacteria**. Gut bacteria are microorganisms that live inside the intestine. Beneficial gut bacteria help to absorb nutrients and vitamins, as well as training the immune system and protecting the system against alien microbes.[31]

Several studies have correlated **reduced gut bacteria** with higher rates of allergies.[32] The use of antibiotics in the first two years of life has been shown to reduce the amount of beneficial bacteria in the gut, in particular those bacteria known as bifidobacteria and bacteroides.[33] Bifidobacteria and bacteroides are beneficial bacteria that help train the body's immune system and a reduction of them can potentially damage the way the body responds to invaders.

Bifidobacteria and bacteroides are amongst a group of beneficial gut bacteria known as **probiotics**. Aside from being found inside a healthy intestine, probiotics can also be found in fermented foods, such as yogurt or sauerkraut. Many of the studies referenced in this section used either probiotics in pill form, or fermented milk (yogurt) for their testing.

Recent studies have indicated that **probiotics may have both a preventative *and* therapeutic effect on the immune system**. Intake of probiotics during infancy has been shown to reduce the likelihood of allergies later in life, as well as reduce symptoms in adults with allergies.[34] The beneficial effect of probiotics for infants may even start as early as conception. For example, one Danish study found that children of women who drank whole milk or ate full fat yogurt during pregnancy had significantly lower rates of hay fever and asthma compared to women who ate low-fat yogurt.[35] On the other hand, low-fat yogurt was directly related to *higher* rates of asthma and allergic rhinitis. This is likely because whole milk and full fat yogurt have more probiotics and usually less artificial sweeteners than low-fat or fat free yogurt.

To put it simply and to go back to our analogy, let's consider probiotics as the immune system's **drill sergeants**. Probiotic drill sergeants teach the special forces, (the IgE antibodies) to develop a healthy immune system in which they are able to recognize true enemy invaders versus benign pollens and foods.

In general, studies indicate that increasing probiotic intake early in life can have a positive effect on preventing allergies and may help reduce lung inflammation and allergic reactions in older allergy sufferers. However, some of the same studies have found that the beneficial effect is limited during periods when pollen counts are high.[36] Furthermore, results have not been uniform. As research is still ongoing it is unclear in what form and in what amounts probiotics may be beneficial, although both bifidobacteria and lactobacilli are the two probiotics considered to be the most helpful in producing good gut bacteria.[37]

In addition to antibiotics, various other factors have been correlated to lower amounts of beneficial gut bacteria, such as cesarean births, having been breastfed, having an older sibling, and growing up in a farm environment. Studies have shown that **cesarean births** (C-section) tend to result in lower amounts of beneficial gut bacteria and *higher* amounts of detrimental gut bacteria than in infants born vaginally.[38] These detrimental bacteria, known as *E. coli* and *C. difficile*, are associated with flu-like symptoms such as bloating, abdominal pain and cramping, diarrhea and even infections.

In birth studies similar to those done on cesarean births, it has been found that children who are **breastfed** exclusively (versus those that have been formula fed or both breastfed and formula fed) have the highest levels of beneficial gut bacteria and the lowest numbers of C. difficile and E. coli.[39]

Having an older sibling also seems to have a positive effect on beneficial gut bacteria. Various studies of teenagers and children have found that having an older sibling corresponded to *lower rates* of allergic rhinitis, whereas those with only a younger sibling were *more likely* to have AR,[40] even more so than those without a younger sibling at all.[41] It has been suggested that having an older sibling has a positive effect on gut bacteria.[42] However, it is not entirely clear *why* this is so, and more research is needed.

A **lack of Vitamin D** has also been correlated with higher rates of allergies. For example, one Finnish study found that children and teenagers with allergies were more likely to have vitamin D deficiency.[43] In keeping with other studies on allergies potentially starting in the womb, it has been found that maternal intake of Vitamin D from foods sources (not supplements) during pregnancy is associated with a reduced risk of allergies and asthma in children. Conversely, studies have shown that Vitamin D taken in the form of supplements during pregnancy and early childhood are actually associated with a *higher risk* of allergies. This suggests that getting Vitamin D from food sources is more beneficial than taking supplements, which can be detrimental to allergies. [44] The relationship between Vitamin D and allergies is still unclear. Whether a lack of Vitamin D is a contributing factor to the development of allergies, or those with allergies happen to have an inability to absorb Vitamin D is not known.

A recent study published in April of 2013 found that probiotics may help to increase Vitamin D absorption.[45] Out of 127 test subjects, those who took Vitamin D along with probiotics were found to have over a 20% increase in absorption of Vitamin D, versus those who took Vitamin D with a placebo. This indicates that a combination of probiotics and Vitamin D could potentially be beneficial for improving immune function. However, much more testing needs to be done to determine if probiotics truly are able to help the absorption of Vitamin D and if probiotics and Vitamin D can help to reduce allergic reactions.

One more significant factor in the development of a healthy immune system with beneficial gut bacteria is **environment**. Numerous studies from a variety of countries around the world have found that people in rural areas have lower rates of allergies than those in urban areas.[46] For example, a recently published study that examined 8,259 children from Switzerland, Austria and Germany found that 4% of non-farm children reported having hay fever, whereas only 1% of farm children reported it.

The higher rates of allergies in urban areas have led to studies on the **protective effects of farming**. It is speculated that the higher numbers of microbes found on farms have a positive effect on training the immune system.[47] Like the other factors mentioned so far, the positive effects of growing up in a farm environment may begin as early as in the womb.[48] Maternal exposure to a variety of farm animals is associated with decreased allergen sensitivity in children. Childhood exposure to a variety of farm animals may also be beneficial for long term allergy protection. For example, a Finnish study found that contact with farm animals in early childhood reduced the risk of allergies, even at age 31.[49] The protective effect was particularly evident in those whose mothers had worked with farm animals during pregnancy. The study also found that having cats and dogs during childhood had a similar protective effect against allergies.

Furthermore, a study of over 18,000 Swedish inhabitants found that the protective effect of growing up on a farm was significantly pronounced later in life. Those who grew up on a farm and were between the ages of 16-30 had a hay fever rate of 19.5%, whereas those from urban areas had a rate of 30.5%.[50]

Another factor associated with rural living and allergies is **pollution and pollen counts**. While it might be assumed that pollen counts are higher in rural areas, where there are more trees and plants, in fact the opposite can be true. Studies have shown that plants in urban areas react more strongly to the higher rates of pollution. For example, both cypress and timothy grass **release more allergens** when they are exposed to high concentrations of nitrogen dioxide and ozone, the chemicals which are released by automobiles and industrial emissions.[51]

Air pollution can actually act as a platform of sorts to transfer allergens and pollens into the respiratory system. Air pollution may also exacerbate allergic symptoms, and can impair the respiratory tract and mucus membranes.[52] Essentially, when the mucus membranes are damaged, it slows down the clearing of mucus and pollen from the system, so the effects of pollen are prolonged.[53] Long term studies in countries with high rates of air pollution, such as China and Turkey, suggest that the effect is cumulative, and long-term exposure to air pollution increases the likelihood of developing allergies.[54]

Unfortunately, some of the most allergenic **plants are producing more allergens and spreading** over greater areas. If the global temperature continues to rise as projected,[55] this trend is only expected to worsen. It has been demonstrated that a temperature rise of only 1-2 degrees Celsius is enough to cause ragweed to produce significantly more pollen, grow faster and flower earlier. [56] Already countries such as Canada,[57] Spain,[58] Greece,[59] Poland,[60] Switzerland,[61] and Denmark[62] have found that pollen seasons for allergens such as birch, ragweed, and oak start earlier, last longer, and have higher pollen counts than in previous years. In the northern town of Thessaloniki in Greece, a study conducted from 1987 – 2005 found that, on average, the pollen concentration in the air *doubled* every 10 years, and for some species it even doubled every 5 years.[63] In a scary estimate of what could happen by the end of the 21st century, in the Iberian Peninsula oak pollen season is expected to start one month earlier, and pollens will increase by 50%.[64] Simulated studies have shown that those in the North American prairies may expect a 60-90% increase in ragweed pollen by the end of the 21st century if temperatures continue to heat up.[65]

So does all this mean you should pack up, move to the country, buy a farm, and drive a solar car?

Well it might not be a bad idea. But in the meantime, there are some things you can do to limit your exposure to other factors that are also implicated in the rising rates of allergies.

Chemical substances such as pesticides, herbicides, fertilizers, chemical cleaners, smoke and solvents such as paint, glues, nail polish and polish remover have all been implicated in aggravating, or even causing, allergic rhinitis. Numerous studies have shown that exposure to chemical pesticides, herbicides and fertilizers are correlated with high rates of AR. Again, this may start as early as in the womb. For example, a recent study of Mexican newborns found pesticide use in the home was a strong predicator of high IgE levels in umbilical cord blood.[66] A US study found high levels of the pesticide compound dichlorophenols in people's urine. The higher the levels of dichlorophenols, the more likelihood there was of food allergies.[67]

Farmers and those who are exposed to pesticides, fertilizers and herbicides have particularly high rates of AR. One recent study of Iowan farmers found that 74% who used commercial pesticides reported at least one episode of hay fever over the course of a year. The high rates were suspected to be a result of pesticide, insecticide and fungicide use.[68] In Crete, Greece, pesticide and herbicide use was significantly associated with higher rates of allergic rhinitis in grape farmers.[69] Furthermore, a US study done on farm workers before and after exposure to pesticides found that exposure was more likely to increase IgE antibodies (the special forces units), and increase skin sensitization; the more exposure, the higher the levels of IgE.[70] By avoiding all use of chemical pesticides, herbicides and fertilizers, you may decrease the likelihood of aggravating existing allergies, as well as preventing them in those around you.

Furthermore, **avoiding foods that have been sprayed with chemicals**, pesticides, herbicides and fungicides may also help to prevent exacerbating and causing allergies. A Canadian study found pesticide residue in the blood of various urban women. In particular, pesticides were found in the umbilical blood and fetuses of pregnant women, most likely due to the women having eaten genetically modified food sprayed with pesticides.[71] If exposure in the air can aggravate allergies, it is not impossible that ingesting them would be just as bad, if not worse.

Since genetically modified foods are most likely to have been sprayed with chemical compounds, it may be safer to look for foods that are either organic or spray-free and non-GMO, meaning that no genetically modified organisms have been used in making them.

Various other types of **indoor air pollutants**, also known as *volatile organic compounds* (VOCs), such as air fresheners, cleaners, new furniture and carpets, and paint may also exacerbate, or even cause, allergies. Numerous studies have shown that exposure to toxic chemicals in products that are frequently used inside the home can cause increased rates of IgE antibodies, food allergies, hay fever, and asthma, as well as an altered immune system.[72] Again, this may begin as early as in the womb. Renovations that involve new paint, wallpaper, PVC flooring, plastic and formaldehyde are also high risk for an increase in allergies, asthma and wheezing. In particular, the use of chemical cleaners has been found to double the odds for children developing persistent wheezing. It may be that long-term exposure to small amounts of chemicals can result in a cumulative effect, continuing to exacerbate symptoms.

Those who live and work in newer homes or buildings where VOC levels are higher may also be at higher risk. Studies have found that those who are exposed to high levels of VOCs in newer buildings often complain of mucus membrane irritation, fatigue, difficulty concentrating and upper respiratory problems.[73]

Second-hand smoke has also been implicated in aggravating allergies. For example, a group of volunteers exposed to second-hand smoke and then ragweed were found to have produced significantly higher levels of IgE and histamines than those who had only been exposed to clean air and ragweed.[74] A whole four days after exposure to tobacco smoke, their IgE levels were 16.6 times higher on average than those with only clean air and ragweed. Nasal histamine levels were 3.3 times higher as well. This strongly suggests that second-hand smoke can aggravate allergies.

It stands to reason, then, that **avoiding VOCs such as chemical cleaners, air fresheners, paints, plastics and cigarette smoke** could help to prevent allergies from not only developing, but from worsening. Consider using organic or natural cleaners, such as vinegar and baking soda based cleaners and non-toxic paint that is free of solvents and VOCs. When possible, opt for glass products instead of plastic and toss those chemical air fresheners that can obstruct your airway and make your skin itch.[75]

What you eat and drink out of may also affect the potential for allergies. Exposure to **Bisphenol A (BPAs)**, a man-made chemical compound used in plastics and food containers, has been shown to correspond to higher rates of allergies in several studies.[76] While Bisphenol A has been banned in infant feeding bottles in some countries,[77] as BPAs have been found in high levels in the urine of infants, it still continues to be used in many canned and boxed food and drink containers around the world. For example, in Taiwan, where BPAs are still allowed in plastic baby bottles, a 2012 Taiwanese study of almost 15,000 children found that the longer the use of plastic feeding bottles for infants with BPAs and other chemicals, the higher the likelihood for allergic rhinitis in the toddler years.[78]

Look for foods that are canned in glass containers or BPA-free cans and bottles to help prevent aggravating or causing allergies. Alternatively, buying fresh, pesticide-free food and cooking, canning, freezing and/or preserving it at home is a safer option.

Another consumable, **Omega 3 fatty acids** from fish, has been suggested to help reduce the risk of allergies. Omega 3s are a group of fatty acids found most commonly in fish oil. For example, a recently published 12 year study of over 3,200 Swedish children found that regular consumption of fish in infancy reduced the risk of allergic rhinitis.[79] Other studies also suggest that the earlier the introduction of fish, the better the preventative benefits.[80] While these studies are relatively new and much more research is needed, there is some suggestion that Omega 3 fatty acids and fish consumption *may* aid in the reduction of allergic sensitization.[81]

Lest you find all this information overwhelming, let's take a moment to recap here and review some of the risk factors and potential preventative measures for hay fever and, by association, oral allergy syndrome.

Risk factors & aggravations for allergies include (in no particular order):

- Genetics (a parent with allergic rhinitis)
- Lack of probiotics in the gut
- Antibiotic use
- C-section birth
- Lack of Vitamin D
- Outdoor air pollution (motor vehicles, industrial emissions, etc)
- Rising global temperature and pollen counts
- Pesticide, fertilizer, herbicide and insecticide exposure (externally and internally)

- Indoor air pollution / volatile organic chemicals (VOCs) such as chemicals, cleaners, paint, new plastic materials, new carpets/flooring, etc.
- Smoke
- Bisphenol A (BPA) exposure

Potential preventative measures and treatments include:

- Immunotherapy (allergy shots or sublingual therapy, i.e. honey infused with pollens)
- Alternative medicine (acupuncture, dietary changes, etc)
- Vaginal birth
- Breastfeeding
- Growing up on a farm/with pets
- Having an older sibling
- Probiotic consumption
- Vitamin D
- Omega 3 consumption
- Reducing exposure to indoor and outdoor air pollution

Furthermore, following the tips in the rest of this chapter for managing OAS and hay fever may help to reduce symptoms and allow your immune system time to recover to some extent.

❧ Guidelines and Tips for Managing OAS ❦

While there is no confirmed treatment at present, there are some guidelines and tips to follow that can be useful for managing OAS. Over the years I've found these methods to reduce some of my own symptoms to both pollens and the foods associated with OAS.

* **Carry epinephrine** (or an epi-pen) if you think you or your child are at risk for anaphylaxis. Ask your doctor for a prescription.

* **Antihistamines** can be helpful for treating symptoms after contact with allergens and foods.

* **Follow a diet** that takes into account your or your child's dietary restrictions.

* **Treat and process** foods to kill the allergen proteins so they can be eaten. Peeling, boiling, microwaving and cooking can destroy the allergens in some foods. (See Chapter 2 for details on this).

* **Avoid foods** that are most offensive and likely to cause severe reactions or anaphylaxis.

* **Read food labels.** Scrutinize ingredient lists for potential sources of allergens. Wheat, soy and nuts are common ingredients associated with OAS that are frequently found in store-bought foods. (See Chapter 2 for hidden sources of wheat and soy).

* **Educate those around you.** Make sure to tell family and friends, and especially caregivers in charge of children with OAS, about allergies and how to avoid contamination. This may include such steps as hand washing and carefully cleaning any surfaces that may have come in to contact with allergy-causing food, or explaining how to administer epinephrine.

* **Don't be shy.** While you may not want to inconvenience friends, family and restaurant staff with your awkward allergies (or potentially be accused of "imagining things" or "being difficult"), keep in mind that your safety is extremely important. Keep a list of things you or your child is allergic to that you can pass on to friends when they're planning dinner parties. It doesn't always make you the favorite dinner guest, but it's better than potentially ruining a party by going into anaphylactic shock at the dinner table.

* **Just say no** to something if you're not sure it's safe. Barbeques, picnics, restaurants, birthdays and dinner parties can be risky business if you don't know exactly what's in everything on the table. Lots of people don't understand the severity of food allergies and if you aren't sure of something's ingredients it's probably safer to avoid it.

* **Carry your own food** if you are going to a public function where food is being served. Bring something along that you know is safe so you or your child won't starve in the event there is nothing for you to eat. Also, your host might not feel as terrible about you going without if you've got something with you to munch on. See Chapter 2 for snack ideas.

* **Manage hay fever** and allergies so that the symptoms are reduced.

❧ Managing an Allergic Reaction ❧

Since reactions can range from extremely mild to severe, from a little itch to the ever-frightening anaphylaxis, it is important to know which allergens are your most reactive and which you should avoid completely. If your throat has swelled, breathing has been constricted, or you've experienced anaphylactic shock, that food should probably be avoided in all forms. However, in the event of a reaction, here are some steps to consider.

* **Drink or eat something,** this can help wash the allergens down from the mouth and throat area, reducing tingling and swelling. Drinking something warm (not scalding) could help to denature the allergen proteins.

* **Take an anti-histamine** if symptoms are strong and unpleasant. Note that these usually take about 30 minutes to work, by which time most symptoms will have dissipated.

* **Relax and rest.** Essentially, it is as if your body is going into battle, and it can be physically draining. If you have gastro-intestinal symptoms, be sure to drink lots of water to stay hydrated.

* **If breathing is restricted** or any symptoms of anaphylaxis are displayed, apply epinephrine immediately and call an ambulance.

❧ Managing Seasonal Allergies in General ❧

Managing hay fever may help to reduce some of the symptoms associated with allergies and OAS, and make hay fever season a little less unpleasant.

* **Keep things clean.** Get rid of dust and pollen by vacuuming regularly and washing floors with vinegar and lemon juice mixed with water. Harsh chemicals may cause further irritation.

* **Keep windows shut** and don't let pollen in to the house.

* **Wash bed sheets in hot water weekly** to rid them of pollens and dust that may have settled.

* **Keep pets at bay.** During peak pollen times pets that have been outdoors can carry in pollens from outside. Keeping them inside is ideal, but otherwise, make sure to wash your hands after touching pets and avoid touching your eyes or face to reduce

the likelihood of pollen entering your nasal passage. Regular bathing of pets helps to remove pollens.

* **Shower regularly** because, like pets, you can track pollens into the house on your clothes and in your hair.

* **Cover bed mattress and pillows** with allergy dust covers that protect against dust mites. I also cover my bed with a sheet during the day which I carefully remove at night. This protects it from pollen that might have filtered in during the day. It also protects it from pets which may have lain on the bed.

* **Air filters are your friend.** Having a good air filter that is changed regularly helps to keep the air clean. There are a variety to consider, such as window screens, furnace filters, and stand-alone units for single rooms.

* **Sinus rinses** can help flush pollens out of sinuses and ease symptoms. Use a netti pot, or a sprayer and salt packages available at the pharmacy.

* **Check the pollen report.** Avoid going outside when the pollen counts are high. Peak times for pollen are in the morning and on windy, dry days.

* **Avoid indoor and outdoor air pollution.** As mentioned in the section on causes of allergies, carbon emissions from vehicles and industrial emissions can aggravate allergies, as can pesticides and fertilizers. Indoor air pollution such as chemical cleaners, paints, etc. may also exacerbate allergies. Keeping a chemical-free home, while difficult, may help to prevent allergy flare-ups.

❧ Managing Exercise: ❦

Food-dependent, exercise-induced anaphylaxis

One rare but important condition to be aware of is food-dependent, exercise-induced anaphylaxis (FDEIA). FDEIA refers to cases in which a person experiences an allergic reaction or even anaphylactic shock while exercising after eating something they are allergic to. Fatalities from FDEIA are extremely rare,[82] but some may experience a range of symptoms and knowing the warning signs can be very helpful. Symptoms typically set in within 30 minutes after exercise is begun and, as the body temperature rises, most often include itching, burning, hives, swelling of the face, throat and tongue, flushing, and difficulty swallowing. In rare and extreme cases, some people may lose of consciousness, experience nausea and anaphylaxis.[83]

FDEIA is fairly unpredictable and not well understood for several reasons. Although one of the earliest cases of anaphylaxis-like symptoms was reported in 1839, research into it is fairly new, with some of the earliest studies being done in the 1980s.[84]

Furthermore, it is unclear who is at risk and to what extent, but *sex and weather may be a factor*. For example, women seem more likely than men to experience FDEIA, with symptoms typically appearing in one's 20's or 30's.[85] Severity of symptoms may fluctuate even for those who have experienced FDEIA. Exercising in high heat and humidity are particularly associated with greater risk of symptoms, as is cold weather to a lesser extent.[86] It does not seem to matter whether the exercise is intense or mild, as both jogging and walking can induce symptoms.

What foods are associated with food-dependent, exercise induced anaphylaxis?

A wide range of both OAS and non-OAS related foods and allergens have been noted as factors in FDEIA. Some of the more common foods associated with exercise-induced anaphylaxis include alcohol, shellfish, tomatoes, peanuts, seeds, cow's milk, and celery.[87] In particular, *wheat* has been known to cause severe reactions prior to exercising, and in 2011 alone several cases of wheat-dependent exercise-induced anaphylactic shock were reported in Japan.[88] Other non-food related items associated with FDEIA include aspirin, non-steroidal anti-inflammatory drugs (NSAIDS), penicillin and antibiotics, and dust mites.[89]

So how does one avoid FDEIA? It is generally advised that people with FDEIA avoid exercise for several hours after eating or taking aspirin and other NSAIDS. Exercising in very warm, humid weather or in the cold should also be avoided.[90] It is important to stop exercising if you experience any of the symptoms described above, as continuing to exercise can cause symptoms to worsen. Carrying epinephrine when exercising and exercising with someone who is aware of your condition and knows how to administer epinephrine is also a good idea.[91]

❧ *Managing Cosmetics Use* ❧

Cosmetics can contain wheat, soy and other OAS-related food oils that can cause allergic reactions. Shampoos, make-up, soap, etc. can all contain hydrolyzed wheat proteins, a compound made with wheat, along with other potential allergens such as soy and almond, sunflower or sesame seed oil.

Hydrolyzed wheat protein and other OAS-related foods have been known to cause allergic reactions ranging from hives and eczema to anaphylaxis when applied topically through the use of cosmetics.[92] For example, in February 2012 a case was reported in which a 16 year old girl with OAS developed severe eczema after using a facial soap that contained hydrolyzed wheat proteins.[93] In 2011, several cases of wheat-dependent exercise-induced anaphylactic shock (explained above in the section on *Managing Exercise*) were reported in Japan after patients were exposed to hydrolyzed wheat protein through their facial soap prior to exercising.[94] Soaps and shampoos, make-up, chap-stick and lotions can contain wheat and soy products, as well as the essential oils of allergenic foods.

It is also important to check for other OAS-related allergens in various cosmetics, essential oils and massage oils, as studies have reported numerous cases of people experiencing contact dermatitis (rashes and hives) after coming in contact with various oils such as almond, sunflower and sesame oil.[95]

☙ *Eating Out* ❧

Eating out can be one of the most difficult things to do with OAS, especially since many restaurants are unaware of the allergy. Most of the suggestions for managing OAS in the earlier section apply to eating out, but here are a few more things I've found helpful for restaurants in particular.

* **When planning to go out** check a restaurant's menu online to get a sense of whether or not you'll find anything to eat.

* **Call ahead** to see if the restaurant can accommodate your allergies, or if they offer an allergy menu. Sometimes if you let a restaurant know you're coming, they can ensure they have specialty items like wheat/gluten free pasta on hand.

* **Go gluten, soy and nut free** if wheat, soy and nuts are problems for you. Gluten is a protein found in wheat and is a common allergy. While restaurant staff may never have heard of OAS, they should be aware of gluten, soy and nut allergies.

* **Beware buckwheat.** Buckwheat is gluten free so it is sometimes found in gluten/wheat free products. However, gluten free does not always mean it is safe for OAS people. Buckwheat is an OAS food and can cause allergic reactions. If you find an item that is gluten free, make sure it is also buckwheat free.

* **Choose cooked or baked dishes** over raw fruit and vegetables. The high heating process denatures the allergen protein in most fruit and vegetables, making them safer for most people to eat.

* **Carry your own food** or eat a small meal ahead of time just in case. For example, I almost always keep a bag of rice cakes in my car for emergencies.

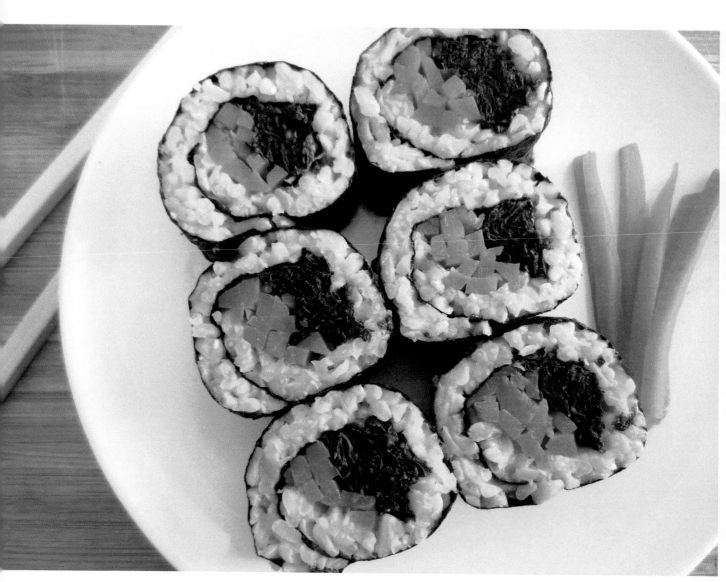

Vegetable Maki Rolls

❧ Chapter 2 ❧

Cooking for OAS

Sometimes sufferers of OAS may feel as if they are allergic to almost everything. This can be particularly frustrating in the case of parents who want to ensure that their kids eat a healthy, balanced diet, but are afraid to feed their kids fresh fruits and vegetables that may cause a bad reaction. This chapter provides information on processing and modifying some of the OAS associated foods so that they may be incorporated back into your diet, as well as a list of foods not commonly associated with OAS. In the case of those foods that can't be modified, such as wheat and soy, in-depth information and alternatives are provided.

It is a good idea to wear non-latex gloves (particularly if allergic to latex) if handling foods you are reactive to. Skin reactions are not uncommon in people with OAS, and you may experience tingling, itchiness, redness, hives, or, in rare cases, shortness of breath and anaphylaxis. Avoid cross-contamination with items like wheat and nuts by keeping food separate in cupboards and clean surfaces with hot soapy water. Some may choose to wear a face mask to avoid airborne particles.

❧ Treating Fruits and Veggies for Safer Consumption ❧

By processing foods at high heats for extended periods of time, the allergen proteins of some allergenic fruits and vegetables are actually destroyed.[96] This is because certain food proteins are *heat labile*, meaning that high heat destroys the allergen proteins. Please note this is not the case for all OAS related foods, nor is it necessarily the case for all proteins within a given piece of fruit. **Nuts, wheat and soy in particular can still cause severe reactions after being heated,** although some people may find that peeled and roasted nuts are more palatable.

Peeling – Removing the peel or waxy outer coating can make it easier for people with allergies to eat some OAS related foods.[97] Several studies have shown that the peels of some fruits, such as apples, peaches and pears, have a higher percentage of allergenicity than the inside core. Although there are still allergen proteins in the pulp of the fruit, the bulk of the allergen proteins are concentrated in the peel or outer coating. At present it doesn't appear that the whole range of OAS related foods has been tested, but some people with milder allergies find that certain fruits and vegetables cause less of a reaction when peeled.

Boiling and Cooking – Studies have shown that many fruits and vegetables that have been processed on high heat for several minutes have significantly reduced allergenicity. [98] As not all proteins in all fruits and vegetables are affected equally, (for example, not all the allergens in celery are heat labile and cooked celery has been known to cause reactions in some, but not others with raw celery allergies)[99] more research needs to be done on specifically which cooked foods are safe, and how much safer. However, many people find that fruits and vegetables that have been cooked or boiled on high heat can be enjoyed without reaction.

Dehydrating – While dehydrated foods may not always have been processed on high heat the same way that canned foods have been, it is possible that even low heat over a long period of time may help break down some of the allergen proteins. It has been suggested that dehydrated foods may cause less of an allergic reaction than fresh fruits or vegetables.[100] However, some people may find that they still react to dehydrated foods that have not been processed on high heat.

Ultimately, many people find that peeling and cooking or boiling foods significantly reduces the possibility of an allergic reactions. For example, canned peaches and pears are less likely to cause tingly lips than fresh ones. Boiled carrots can make a great salad, whereas fresh ones may cause cramps. The recipes in this book make use of cooked or canned fruits and vegetables, as well as various fruits and vegetables not commonly associated with oral allergy syndrome. It is always a good idea, however, to test foods with an oral challenge in the presence of a medical professional if there is any chance of a severe reaction.

❧ The "Right Ingredients" ❦

There are several things to be aware of when choosing ingredients. Ingredients free of chemicals can go a long way to preventing further aggravation of your already highly-alert system. When buying either fresh or canned foods, look for **organic or spray free**, whenever possible (spray-free, or 'cide-free meaning they are free of pesticides, herbicides, fertilizers and fungicides). Organic does not always mean more expensive, and many farmers markets and local community supported agriculture (CSA) programs work with farmers who are organic or use organic practices but are not certified, so you can find chemical free produce cheap. Furthermore, spending more on chemical free and organic produce now could potentially save big money on health problems in the long run.

Secondly, I strongly suggest **avoiding fruits and vegetables canned in corn syrup**. Corn syrup is made with genetically modified organisms (GMOs) which are, as mentioned earlier, heavily sprayed with chemical fertilizers, insecticides, and herbicides that may further unbalance the system. Most fruits and veggies can be found canned in pear juice, pineapple juice, apple juice or in their own juices. Alternatively, canning fruits and vegetables at home following safe practices can ensure their safety.

On that note, you may also choose to **avoid products made with corn**, unless they are organic or non-GMO. For example, baking powder and powdered icing sugar often contain corn starch. Look for organic, GMO-free or corn-free products to avoid ingesting chemicals.

As mentioned in the first chapter under *What Causes Allergies*, it may help to avoid foods canned in **Bisphenol A (BPA) free cans**. BPA is the chemical compound used to line food and drink containers, and has been banned from use in baby bottle and packaging in several countries due to controversial studies that found BPA in human urine. A correlation between BPA found in drinking water and asthma and allergic sensitivities has been found.[101]

❧ Wheat Allergies vs Celiac Disease ☙
& Non-Celiac Gluten Intolerance

Wheat is high on the list of foods that cross-reacts with birch pollen. Scientists are really just beginning to classify the various different types of issues and allergies associated with wheat and gluten, a protein found in wheat. In recent years there has been much to-do about gluten and wheat allergies and celiac disease. Having a wheat allergy does not necessarily mean that you have a gluten sensitivity, or celiac disease. Furthermore, there are various types of wheat allergies, such as baker's asthma, or exercise-induced anaphylaxis. Knowing the differences between wheat allergies, gluten intolerance, or celiac disease can help you to better understand your own allergies and reactions.

❧ Celiac disease ❦

Celiac, or coeliac disease, is a genetic intolerance to gluten. Gluten is a binding agent in commercial wheat products, including barley and rye. For those with celiac disease, exposure to gluten can cause severe reactions. Stomach upset, malaise, fatigue, painful breakouts and cysts, weight gain or loss and the inability to absorb nutrients are only some of the reactions of celiac sufferers. Celiac disease can be tested for through blood work or an endoscopy. Left untreated, celiac disease can cause severe and sometimes permanent damage to the intestine and lead to a wide variety of other illnesses as a result of malabsorption of vitamins, nutrients and calories. At least 1% of the population has CD, however, there are likely many more undiagnosed.[102]

❧ Gluten intolerance or sensitivity: ❦
a.k.a. *non-celiac gluten sensitivity (NCGS)*

Those with NCGS suffer essentially the same symptoms of celiac disease, along with numbness in the legs, arms or fingers and joint pain, but generally do not appear to have the permanent intestinal damage of those with celiac disease. At present gluten intolerance is usually determined through an elimination diet in which any source of gluten is removed from the diet for a significant period of time, then added back in to determine the reaction. It is unknown what percentage of the population suffers from NCGS as many cases go undiagnosed and undocumented.

❧ Wheat allergy ❦

Wheat allergies usually cause an immediate, histamine response to wheat, often with symptoms similar to hay fever such as swelling, stuffy nose, hives, shortness of breath or even anaphylaxis. It may also cause stomach upset and indigestion. Wheat allergies are often linked to OAS and birch pollen allergies. Some, however, are attributed to baker's asthma which affects those who are in constant contact with wheat.

❧ Baker's asthma ❦

Baker's asthma is a type of wheat allergy that has been known since the time of the Ancient Romans. This type of allergy seems to develop over time after constant exposure to wheat. According to a Polish study, signs of respiratory problems due to baker's asthma were observed in 4.2% of bakery apprentices after only one year and in 8.6% after two years.[103]

In the end, despite these biological differences, those with wheat allergies, NCGS or celiac disease are best off following a wheat and gluten free diet. Wheat is in a surprising number of different types of food, and knowing some of the main hidden sources of wheat can help you to avoid accidentally eating them.

⮵ Hidden sources of wheat ⮷

- Beer
- Bouillon cubes
- Breads
- Breakfast cereals
- Bulgur
- Bran
- Candy, cakes and muffins
- Condiments, such as ketchup
- Cookies
- Couscous
- Crackers
- Dairy products, such as ice cream
- Durum Wheat-]
- Farina
- Gelatinized starch
- Gravy
- Hot dogs
- Hydrolyzed vegetable protein Ice cream
- Jelly beans
- Kamut
- Licorice
- Malt
- Meat products, such as hot dogs or cold cuts
- Modified food starch
- Monosodium glutamate (MSG)
- Natural flavorings
- Pasta
- Processed meats
- Semolina
- Soup mixes and broth (vegetable or meat)
- Soy sauce
- Spelt
- Vegetable gum
- Vegetable starch
- Wheat bran, germ, or starch
- Cosmetics

If you have a wheat allergy, you may also be allergic to other grains with similar proteins. These related grains include:

- Barley
- Bulgur
- Kamut
- Oat
- Rye
- Semolina
- Spelt

❧ Wheat and Gluten Free Flours Explained ❦

Gluten is a protein that acts as a binding agent in wheat flour and other related flours. Baking wheat free, and therefore gluten free, generally requires a combination of flours to achieve a similar texture and consistency to glutinous wheat flour. Other ingredients, such as xanthan or guar gum, flaxmeal, eggs and apple cider vinegar are often added to help bind flours and give "lift" to baked goods.

Gluten free (GF) flours and baking can be pretty intimidating if you've only ever had to decide between whole wheat or white bread. Some gluten free flours can also be expensive and hard to find, although this is improving almost daily. The ones used in this book are some of the most common and readily available in many supermarkets and health food stores.

The below table lists some common GF flours and their properties; not all of them are called for in this book and *not all of them are necessarily OAS friendly*. For example, if you are allergic to almonds, peas, or beans you should probably avoid those flours. Another flour to be aware of is buckwheat flour. Although buckwheat is gluten free and technically not "wheat," buckwheat can cause an allergic reaction due to cross pollination with birch pollen and latex. These flours are generally avoided in this book anyway, with the exception of chickpea flour, which is used in *Chickpea Flatbread (Page 76)*.

As for storing GF flours, it is a good idea to keep them in the fridge or freezer to prevent spoilage in warm temperatures, unless using flours regularly. Xanthan gum and guar gum should always be refrigerated as they are expensive and spoil quickly if left in the cupboard.

Some Common Gluten & Wheat Free Flours

Almond Flour	A heavy, nutrient rich flour used in combination with others. High in protein and calories.
Amaranth	From the small amaranth grain, and not unlike millet and quinoa. Slightly nutty and works well in combination with other flours in baked goods.
Arrowroot	A starch used to thicken sauces; it can be used instead of cornstarch, potato or tapioca starch in baked goods.

Brown Rice Flour	Made from brown rice, a common base for baked goods and used in combination with other flours. Good nutrient content.
Buckwheat Flour	Made from ground, unroasted buckwheat groats. Despite the "wheat" in the title, buckwheat is gluten free. It has a slightly nutty flavour and is nutritious.
Chickpea flour a.k.a. garbanzo bean flour	Nutty flavour, often combined with other flours. Found in health food stores and East Indian markets or the ethnic section of supermarkets.
Coconut Flour	A dense, nutritious flour generally used in small amounts with several eggs to leaven.
Corn flour	Milled from corn, can be used in baked goods mixed with other flours.
Cornmeal	Coarsely ground corn. Good for polenta and cornbread and mixed with other flours in baked goods. Look for organic cornmeal.
Cornstarch	Used to leaven baked goods and thicken soups and sauces. Can generally be replaced by tapioca or arrowroot starch in baked goods.
Flaxmeal:	Made from ground flax seed. Used in GF baking to bind flours together; 1 Tbsp flaxmeal combined with 3 Tbsp water can replace eggs as a binder in most baked goods. *Note that the baked goods often will not rise as high without the lightness of eggs, and can have a slightly gummy texture.
Guar Gum:	Used to bind GF flours together in lieu of gluten, and can be used instead of xanthan gum. Expensive, but usually only used in small amounts so it will last a long time. Keep refrigerated.
Millet flour:	Creamy colour and texture with a mild flavour, millet flour works nicely in baked goods in combination with other flours, providing nutrients and fibre.
Potato Flour:	Not to be confused with potato starch, potato flour has a strong potato flavour and is very heavy. It is rarely called for in baked goods but it is very important to differentiate between potato flour and potato starch.

45

Potato Starch: Used as a "glue" for GF baked goods, mix well with other flours as it can get lumpy.

Pea Flour: Usually made from yellow or green peas, but without the "pea taste" when combined with other flours in baked goods. Good source of nutrients. Usually found by mail order or in ethnic markets.

Quinoa Flour Derived from quinoa grain. High protein content, best used in combination with other grains to prevent heaviness.

Sorghum Flour Sorghum is a nutritious base for GF baked goods, used in combination with starches. One of the closest to regular wheat flour.

Soy Flour Heavy and nutritious, can be used in small amounts in combination with other flours.

Sweet Rice Flour a.k.a. Glutinous Rice Flour Does not actually contain gluten despite its name; it is made from sticky rice and works well in small amounts to keep baked goods moist. It can be found in Asian markets, the ethnic section of supermarkets and natural food stores.

Tapioca Starch a.k.a. Tapioca Flour Helps to bind baked goods. Found in health food stores, supermarkets and Asian markets or ethnic section of supermarkets. Good substitute for cornstarch in baked goods and for thickening sauces.

White Rice Flour Made from ground white rice and common in GF baking, although less nutritious than brown rice flour. Not the same as sweet rice flour.

Xanthan Gum Used in small amounts to replace gluten. it aids in binding baked goods and providing structure, so baked goods don't crumble. Use ¼ tsp to 1 c flour for cakes, and ¼ - ½ tsp per cup of flour for breads, muffins and cookies. Guar gum can generally be used in place of xanthan. Keep xanthan gum refrigerated. Note that some xanthan gums are derived from corn and may contain trace amounts of corn. Look for corn-free xanthan gums to avoid contamination.

❧ Hidden Sources of Soy ❧

Soy, like wheat, can be difficult to avoid. Soy and processed soy products can be found in a wide variety of non-food and food products.

Non-food products that may contain soy or processed soy include:

- Adhesives
- Artificial fire logs
- Blankets
- Body lotions and creams
- Candles
- Carpet backing
- Cleaning products
- Cosmetics
- Crib mattresses
- Enamel paints
- Fabric finishes
- Fabrics
- Fertilizers
- Flooring materials
- Hand sanitizer
- Inks and Toners
- Lotion
- Lubricants
- Medications, vitamins, and supplements
- Modeling dough
- Nitroglycerine
- Paper
- Pet food
- Printing inks
- Puzzles, games, or board books printed with soy-based inks
- Shampoo and conditioner
- Soaps
- Stuffed animal filling

Food products that may contain soy or processed soy include:

- Asian cuisine
- Baby formula and foods
- Baked goods and baking mixes
- Bean curd
- Bouillon cubes
- Breakfast Cereals
- Cakes
- Candy and Chocolate
- Canned or packaged soups
- Canned tuna and fish
- Cereal
- Chicken broth
- Cooking oils
- Crackers
- Deli meats
- Edamame (soybeans)
- Energy and nutrition bars
- Gravy
- Guar gum
- Gum arabic
- Hot dogs

- Hydrolyzed plant protein (HPP) or hydrolyzed vegetable protein (HVP)
- Hydrolyzed soy protein (HSP)
- Imitation dairy foods, i.e. soy milk, vegan cheese or ice cream
- Margarine
- Mayonnaise
- Miso (fermented soybean paste)
- Meat products with spices and fillers, i.e. burgers or sausages
- Mono- and di-glycerides
- MSG (monosodium glutamate)
- Natural flavoring
- Nutrition supplements (vitamins)
- Peanut butter and substitutes
- Protein powders
- Salad dressings
- Sauces, gravies, and soups
- Seasoning salt
- Shoyu
- Smoothies
- Soy lecithin
- Soy products (cheese, grits, milk, nuts, sprouts, yogurt, ice cream, pasta)
- Soy sauce
- Soybean (curds, granules, sprouts)
- Soybean oil
- Stabilizer
- Tamari
- Tempeh
- Teriyaki sauce
- Textured vegetable protein (TVP)
- Thickener
- Tofu
- Vegetable gum, starch, shortening, or oil
- Vegetarian meat substitutes, i.e. veggie burgers, imitation meat patties, lunch meats, ground meat, bacon bits, etc.

Eating In & Substitutions

The following sections involve information on cooking safely at home, suggestions for meals, and ways to substitute and incorporate fruits and vegetables based on your individual dietary restrictions.

Basic meal suggestions for OAS

You can find many snack and meal suggestions throughout the recipe chapters, but here are a few suggestions for basic meal ideas to help guide you in meal planning.

- Stir fries with rice, quinoa, millet, brown rice noodles or vermicelli noodles, using steamed greens and cooked vegetables
- Baked vegetable casseroles
- Soups with gluten/wheat-free noodles or rice and boiled vegetables

- Pastas with cooked or boiled vegetables
- Meal sized salads with steamed greens, rice noodles and boiled fruit purées as dressing
- Baked and steamed vegetables over rice, quinoa or millet

☙ **Snacking suggestions** ❧

- Store-bought rice cakes
- Fruit roll-ups (see *Fruit Leather*)
- Gluten free crackers (see *Brown Rice Crackers*)
- Smoothies made with cooked/boiled/canned fruits (see *Egyptian Yogurt Smoothie* and *Green Tea Pear Smoothie*)
- Fruit salads made with canned fruits
- Use cooked fruit sauce instead of syrup for desserts and pancakes
- Make salad dressings out of cooked fruit purees (see recipes in *Salads & Dressings*)
- Popsicles made from boiled, pureed fruit (see *Rocket Pops* and *Purple Popsicles)*
- Baked breads, rolls and cakes (see recipes in the *Breads & Baked Goods* and *Desserts* chapters)

Some fruits, vegetables and herbs not commonly associated with OAS*

* Artichokes
* Asparagus
* Basil
* Beets
* Blueberries
* Bok choy (and other Asian cabbages)
* Coconut
* Garlic
* Ginger
* Grapes
* Kale
* Leeks
* Mushrooms
* Nori (seaweed)
* Okra
* Onion
* Papaya
* Pineapple
* Radish
* Rhubarb
* Sweet Potato
* Swiss chard
* Spinach
* Turnip
* Water chestnut

* Please note that this list is not definitive, and does not mean some people do not have allergies to these foods, only that OAS related reactions have not been commonly recorded.

∾ *Making Fruit & Vegetable Purées & Substitutions* ∾

Fruit and vegetable purées for use in smoothies, baked goods and sauces can easily be made at home. By following these basic directions, you can avoid buying canned, store-bought purées with questionable ingredients and unsafe packaging. The method you use will depend on the type of fruit or vegetable, but in general, most fruit and vegetables can be washed, peeled, deseeded and boiled in a pot of large water. Cook for 15-20 minutes, until soft. Drain, add to a food processor or blender, or use a hand blender to purée, adding water by the tablespoon if necessary for a smooth consistency.

Softer fruits, such as apples, peaches, pears and berries, and soft vegetables such as spinach, may also be peeled, cored, chopped, and cooked down with small amounts of water added as needed to prevent burning. Cook for 10-20 minutes, until thoroughly softened. If not already puréed by the cooking process, remove to a food processor or blender, or use a hand blender to purée, adding water by the tablespoon if necessary to make a smooth consistency.

Harder vegetables, like sweet potatoes, squash and beets can be roasted rather than boiling, if desired. Roasting can bring out a depth of flavour and juiciness in the vegetables otherwise lost through boiling. For smaller vegetables like beets, bake whole; for larger vegetables like squashes, cut in half. Arrange in a baking dish, cover with tin foil or fitted cover and bake 20 minutes – 1¼ hours at 400F, until thoroughly soft. Cool and peel. Blend in a food processor or blender, or using a hand blender to purée, adding water by the tablespoon if necessary to make a smooth paste.

Excess purée can be frozen in freezer safe containers for later use. Or pour into ice cube trays and remove to freezer bags or containers once frozen. One ice cube equals approximately two tablespoons, so eight ice cubes will yield one cup of purée.

Many of the recipes in this book make use of purées such as applesauce, carrot or sweet potato. In general, however, purées are interchangeable, so feel free to substitute based on your specific allergies. For example, if you know that you cannot have cooked applesauce, but cooked pears are ok, substitute pear purée for applesauce. Or use sweet potato, cantaloupe or beets instead of carrot. Get creative!

The flavour of fruits and vegetables are often undetectable in baked goods, so there's plenty of room to experiment with different fruits and vegetables.

In most typical recipes, fruit or vegetable purées can be used to replace up to half the fat and/or sugar. If replacing sugar with purée, cut back on other liquids roughly proportionately. For example, if a recipe calls for ½ cup sugar and 1 cup milk, try using ¼ cup sugar, ¼ cup purée and ¾ cup milk.

The recipes in this book call for either honey or brown sugar. Some people with OAS may react to raw honey, but may be ok with processed, boiled or baked honey. If in doubt, brown sugar can be used instead. The recipes in this book have not been tested using maple syrup or stevia, a natural powdered sweetener, but either may be a suitable replacement in small amounts.

❧ *Making Seed & Nut Butters* ❧

While not called for in this book, knowing how to make your own seed and nut butters can be extremely useful for those with allergies to various nuts and seeds. It's not always easy or cost-effective to find alternative spreads in store, but it is very simple to make them at home, and you can easily customize them based on your own individual restrictions. *Note that if you are allergic to a seed or nut raw, you may still react to them even after roasting so it's best to avoid using any seed or nut you react to.* Some people, however, do find that roasting makes some nuts more palatable. If there is any doubt, check with a doctor before trying these.

Seeds and nuts that can be used to make butter include: almonds, brazil nuts, cashews, coconut flakes (unsweetened), chestnuts, flax, hazelnuts, hemp seeds, macadamia, peanuts, pecans, pine nuts, sesame, sunflower, and pumpkin seeds.

The basic formula for making seed or nut butter is as follows:

1 c nuts or seeds
1-2 Tbsp olive or coconut oil in liquid form
1-2 Tbsp organic brown sugar, honey or maple syrup
Pinch of salt

1) Preheat oven to 350F. Spread 1 cup of nuts or seeds on a baking sheet and bake for 5-10 minutes until browned, turning halfway through. (This step is optional,

but provides a lovely flavour and, as mentioned above, some may find roasted nuts safer to eat)

2) In a food processor, whirl seeds or nuts for 10 minutes, until they have broken down and become more paste-like.

3) Add 1 tablespoon olive or coconut oil, 1 tablespoon honey, sugar or maple syrup and a pinch of salt. Continue to process another 5-10 minutes, until a smooth consistency is achieved. Adjust oil and sweetener to taste. Keep in a sealed container in the fridge for up to 2 weeks.

Get creative! Experiment with cocoa, cinnamon, or other spices to make different flavours like chocolate or pumpkin spice butter.

❧ On Cooking Lettuces ❦

Salads are considered a staple health food for many people with allergies. However, lettuce and other greens may cause allergic reactions for some as many greens are related to birch, cypress, latex, mugwort and grass pollens. There have been documented cases of hives, breathing difficulties, stomach upset and even anaphylaxis in people with OAS who had handled or ingested lettuce.[104] Although there have been almost no documented cases of reactions, mustard greens, kale and watercress are all part of the Brassicaceae, or mustard family, which is associated with cypress pollen. In raw form, these may cause itching, hives and gastro-intestinal distress. The salad recipes in this book avoid using raw lettuces and instead recommend steaming, sautéing, or cooking various different greens to help reduce their allergenicity. In recipes that call for steaming, you may also sauté or boil the greens. Alternatives to raw lettuce that are good cooked include kale, Swiss chard and mustard greens. Kale is also extremely high in nutrients and vitamins, so steamed, sautéed or cooked kale makes a healthy alternative to raw lettuce.

For more on lettuce allergies, check out my article "Allergic to Lettuce?!" here: http://www.poorandglutenfree.blogspot.com/2012/11/allergic-to-lettuce.html

On Rice Allergies

Although not common, some people can develop allergies to rice. It has very recently been discovered that rice and peaches share a protein, and that rice allergies can arise in those with peach allergies.[105] It has also been found in at least one case in a man with baker's asthma / wheat allergies, who developed hives and wheezing after contact with rice and products with rice flour.[106] Rice and wheat, like rice and peaches, share a common reactive protein. In rare cases it has been found to cause anaphylaxis.[107] If rice or rice flour is a problem for you, try substituting cooked rice or rice noodles with quinoa and millet, and quinoa flour noodles. Instead of rice flour, try sorghum flour in recipes, as the two are similar. Instead of Asian rice noodles, try bean thread or sweet potato noodles.

❧ Chapter 3: Breakfasts ❧

With a little preparation some of the best breakfasts - pancakes, crepes and even fruit and vegetable smoothies - can still be had despite OAS. All of the recipes in this chapter offer delicious ways to sneak in some extra nutrition.

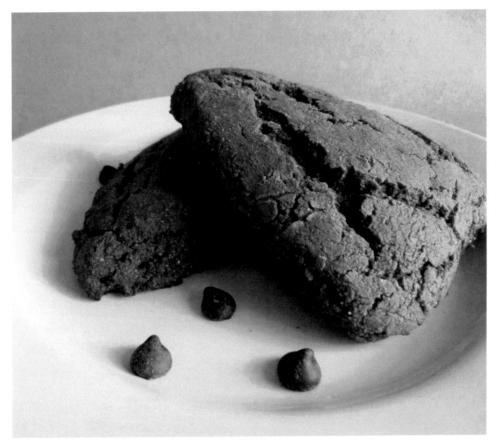

Chocolate Carrot Scones

In this chapter:

Egyptian Yogurt Smoothie

This smoothie is inspired by a yogurt drink I used to sip at a café in Cairo when I once spent a few months studying there. It's a great way to get probiotics.

Makes approximately 1½ cups

1 c organic yogurt

½ c applesauce, puréed peaches or pears

1 Tbsp honey or brown sugar (optional)

⅛ tsp cinnamon

1. In a cup, mix yogurt, applesauce and honey together. Sprinkle with cinnamon and serve.

Green Tea Pear Smoothie

Many people with OAS miss fruit smoothies. Cooked or canned fruit can make easy, enjoyable smoothies packed with healthy goodness.

Makes approximately 4 cups

1 pear or 1-15oz can of pears*

1 c kale leaves, stems removed

¼ tsp vanilla

½" slice ginger, peeled

1 c chilled green tea water

1 Tbsp lemon juice

1. If using raw pear, quarter, core and peel it. In a small pot, cover pear and kale with water and boil 7-10 minutes, until soft.

2. In a blender or food processor, blend together all ingredients until smooth.

* Remaining canned liquid can be used to flavour yogurt, smoothies or salad dressings.

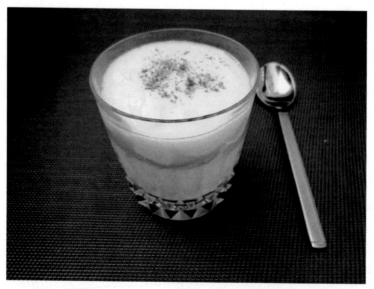

Millet Porridge Mash-Up

A filling and nourishing breakfast, this porridge is also flexible. Add and remove fruit and seasonings as desired, so it's a different breakfast every time. Fruit purées and canned or dried fruit make great additions! **Makes approximately 1 ½ cups**

¼ c millet flour

2 Tbsp raisins or dried cranberries

½ c milk (cow, rice, or coconut, etc.)

½ c water

Pinch of salt

¼ tsp cinnamon

¼ tsp vanilla

2 Tbsp applesauce, puréed peaches or pears

Maple syrup, honey or brown sugar to taste

Top with blueberries or canned fruit slices

1. In a small saucepan, heat millet, raisins or cranberries, milk, water and salt over medium heat. Cook until thick and smooth, approximately 10 minutes, stirring occasionally.

2. Add in cinnamon, vanilla, applesauce, sweeteners and fruit as desired.

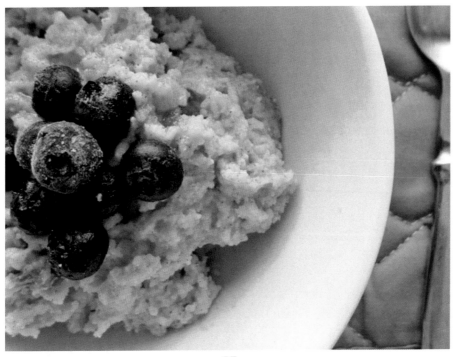

Blueberry Chai Pancakes

Nothing says Sunday morning like a giant stack of chai flavoured blueberry pancakes. They smell heavenly and taste even better. These freeze well between sheets of waxed paper and can be reheated in the oven or microwave.

Makes about 15 pancakes

1¼ c milk (cow, rice, or coconut, etc.)	1 c brown rice flour
1 chai tea bag	½ c tapioca starch
1 egg	3 tsp baking powder
1 tsp vanilla extract	1 tsp baking soda
1 Tbsp oil (olive or melted coconut oil) + more for frying	½ tsp salt
2 Tbsp maple syrup, honey, or sugar	Approximately 1 c blueberries
1 tsp apple cider vinegar	

1. Heat milk over medium heat. Remove from heat and steep chai tea bag for 10 minutes. Bring chai milk to room temperature.

2. In a bowl, whisk chai milk, egg, vanilla, oil, sweetener and cider vinegar until frothy. Beat in dry ingredients to make a smooth batter. Let rest 10 minutes.

3. Heat an oiled skillet over medium heat. Pour batter in skillet in ¼ cups. Add 3-5 blueberries per pancake. Cook until batter bubbles and takes on a dry appearance around the edges. Flip and cook until browned on both sides.

* **Hint:** For whatever reason, the first pancake often ends up messy. It is best to pour a small amount of batter in the pan to test the heat and discard (or eat) the mangled pancake.

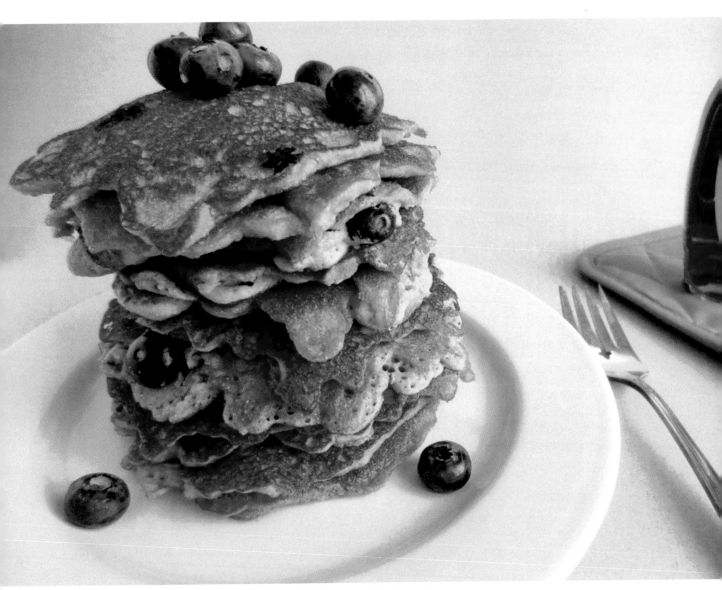

Wheat-Free Blueberry Chai Pancakes

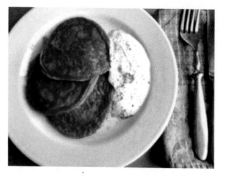

Carrot Cake Pancakes

Using cooked and puréed carrots can make for a tasty and healthy pancake. The carrots add a lovely golden hue to this sweet breakfast treat. These freeze well between sheets of wax paper and can be reheated in the microwave or oven.

Makes approximately 12 pancakes

1 c brown rice flour

½ c tapioca starch

2 tsp baking powder

1-2 Tbsp brown sugar

½ tsp salt

½ tsp ground cinnamon

⅛ tsp ground nutmeg

⅛ tsp ground ginger

1 egg or 1 Tbsp ground flax mixed with 2 Tbsp water

1 c cooked and puréed carrots or sweet potato*

¾ c milk (cow, rice, or coconut, etc.)

2 Tbsp coconut or olive oil

Oil for frying

Heat an electric skillet or pan on medium-high heat.

1. Sift the dry ingredients together in a large bowl. Mix well.

2. Add the egg, carrot, milk, and oil and mix until smooth.

3. Drizzle some oil on a skillet heated over medium heat. Pour batter into pan and cook until batter bubbles and bottom is browned. Flip and cook until browned on both sides. Serve with yogurt, sour cream, maple syrup or fruit compote and sprinkle with cinnamon.

* For the carrot purée, use either 1 can of carrots, or boil several peeled carrots for 15 minutes until soft, then purée in a food processor, adding water as needed to make smooth.

* **Hint:** For whatever reason, the first pancake often ends up messy. It is best to pour a small amount of batter in the pan to test the heat and discard (or eat) the mangled pancake.

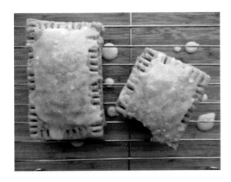

Peach Breakfast Pies (Mock Pop Tart)

Commercial breakfast tarts and pies are often full of sugar and corn syrup, and contain more unnatural ingredients than fruit, even though fruit alone is sweet enough. Substitute apples, pears, blueberries or any other fruit for peaches and make a different breakfast pie every time. **Makes 6-8 fruit pies**

1 batch *Pie Crust*, chilled (*Page 122*)	¼ tsp vanilla
2 peaches or canned equivalent, peeled and finely diced*	1 Tbsp brown sugar, honey or maple syrup (optional)
¼ tsp cinnamon	Icing:
½ tsp lemon juice	1⅓ c icing sugar
1 Tbsp tapioca starch	3-4 Tbsp lemon juice

1. In a saucepot over medium heat, cook diced peaches with cinnamon, lemon juice and starch until soft and sticky, about 10 minutes. Add water by the tablespoon as necessary to prevent burning. Remove from heat and stir in vanilla and sugar.

2. Between two sheets of waxed paper, or on a surface sprinkled with rice flour, roll out pie dough approximately 1/8" thick. Cut into rectangles, roughly the size of a playing card. Scoop approximately 2 tablespoons peach filling into the centre and spread evenly, up to 1/4" from edges. With a wet finger, dampen the edges and cover with another rectangle of dough. Pinch edges or press with a fork to seal. Repeat with remaining dough, re-rolling as necessary. Prick top with a fork to allow steam to escape. If dough becomes too pliable or sticky, chill for 5 minutes.

3. Preheat oven to 350F, oil a baking sheet and cover with parchment paper. Bake breakfast pies on the sheet for approximately 20 minutes, until pie crust is firm but pliable. Cool on a cooling rack.

4. Mix icing sugar and lemon juice together, adding lemon juice as needed to make a smooth icing. Drizzle or spread over cooled pies.

*If using canned fruit, look for fruit canned in pear juice, not corn syrup or sugar. Reserve juice and use to sweeten smoothies, yogurt or salad dressings.

Millet Pancakes

Light and fluffy with a hint of spice, millet flour makes for nutty, healthy pancakes.
Makes approximately 10 pancakes

1 c millet flour	1 egg, beaten
1½ tsp baking soda	5 Tbsp applesauce or cooked pear purée
½ tsp salt	1 Tbsp maple syrup, honey or sugar
½ tsp cinnamon	½ tsp vanilla
⅛ tsp cloves	¼ - ½ c water
	Olive or coconut oil for frying

Heat approximately 1 Tbsp oil in a large skillet over medium heat

1. Sift dry ingredients together.

2. Beat egg, applesauce, maple syrup and vanilla together in a large bowl with ¼ c of the water and blend into dry ingredients until a smooth batter is created. Add more water by the tablespoon as needed. Let batter rest 5 minutes.

3. Pour approximately ¼ cup of batter into the skillet to create pancakes and fry until the batter bubbles, edges appear dry and bottom is browned. Flip and fry on the other side until browned. Repeat with the rest of the batter, adding oil as needed.

*Hint: The first pancake can often end up a bit messy. It is best to pour a small amount of batter in the pan to test the heat and discard (or eat) the mangled pancake.

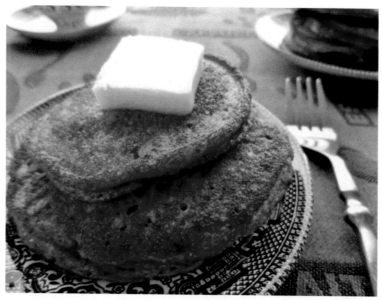

Chocolate Crepes

It doesn't get much better than chocolate crepes for breakfast, or dessert. Serve them with fruit purée, canned fruit, drizzled with chocolate, sprinkled with powdered sugar or whipped cream. **Makes 12 - 6½" crepes**

2 Tbsp cocoa powder	2 eggs, beaten
½ c tapioca starch	1⅓ c milk (cow, rice, or coconut, etc.)
½ c flour (garbanzo bean, sorghum or brown rice flour)	2 Tbsp oil or melted butter
3 Tbsp sugar	
Pinch of salt	

1. Sift together cocoa, starch, flour, sugar and salt. Blend.

2. Whisk eggs and milk into the dry ingredients until smooth.

3. Heat a 6½" cast iron or non-stick skillet over medium heat. Pour a thin layer of batter and swirl to spread evenly. Cover with a tight-fitting lid and cook for 2-3 minutes, until edges begin to curl up. Remove lid and cook another 1-2 minutes, until the crepe begins to look dry. Flip and cook another 2-3 minutes, until both sides are browned. Repeat.

These keep for 2-3 days in the fridge.

*Hint: Like pancakes, the first crepe often ends up messy. It is best to pour a small amount of batter in the pan to test the heat and discard (or eat) the mangled crepe.

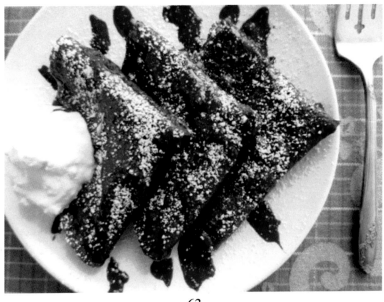

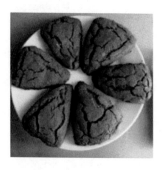

Sweet Potato Chocolate Scones

These can also be made with other types of veggie purées, like squash, pumpkin, or carrots. Substitute raisins or cacao nibs for chocolate chips, if desired. These freeze well and can be reheated in the microwave or left on the counter to thaw.

Servings: 8 large scones

½ c millet flour

½ c tapioca starch

¾ c brown rice flour

¼ c cocoa

½ Tbsp baking powder

¼ tsp baking soda

8 Tbsp butter (or vegan alternative), chilled and sliced in chunks

Extra tapioca flour for dusting

½ cup puréed sweet potato*

3 Tbsp water or yogurt

⅓ c honey or organic brown sugar

1 tsp vanilla

1 Tbsp flax meal mixed with 2 Tbsp water (or 1 egg)

<u>Optional</u>: ¼ c chocolate chips or cacao nibs

Preheat oven to 400F. Spray a cookie sheet with oil and line with parchment paper.

1. Sift flours, cocoa, baking powder, and soda together in the bowl of a food processor. Pulse flours together with the sliced butter until butter is in pea sized chunks. Alternatively, without a food processor, cut the butter into the flour mix using a pastry knife or two knives until crumbly.

2. In a separate bowl, mix the wet ingredients until blended. Add to the dry ingredients and pulse or mix until just combined, avoid over-mixing. If using cacao nibs or chocolate chips, fold them in to the dough very gently.

3. On a lightly floured surface, turn out dough and shape it into a round about 3/4" high and 7" wide. Using a sharp knife, slice into 8 triangles. Arrange slices on baking sheet and bake for 15-17 minutes until firm. Remove to a cooling rack to cool. If desired, drizzle with melted chocolate.

* To make puréed sweet potato, use either canned sweet potato, or peel, dice and boil one medium-sized sweet 10 minutes until soft, then mash.

Green Eggs, No Ham

Personally I'm of the opinion that it's not really a breakfast without eggs, so I actually have some version of this several times a week.

Serves 2

2 eggs, scrambled

½ tsp dried dill or oregano

¼ c EACH chopped green and red peppers

6 cherry tomatoes, halved or quartered depending on size

1½ c Swiss chard leaves, stems removed and loosely chopped

Oil for frying

Salt and pepper to taste

<u>Optional:</u> replace dill with paprika or turmeric, replace chard with spinach or kale, add mushrooms or thinly sliced onion, fresh dill to garnish

1. Scramble eggs with dill in a bowl.

2. Heat 1 Tbsp oil in a medium-sized skillet over medium heat. Sauté peppers for 2 minutes, until slightly softened. Add tomatoes and cook another 2 minutes to soften. Add chard leaves and cook another 2 minutes, until wilted, but not brown.

3. Pour eggs over vegetables and cook 2-3 minutes, stirring to scramble and cook evenly until eggs are firm and not glossy. Remove from heat and serve with salt and pepper.

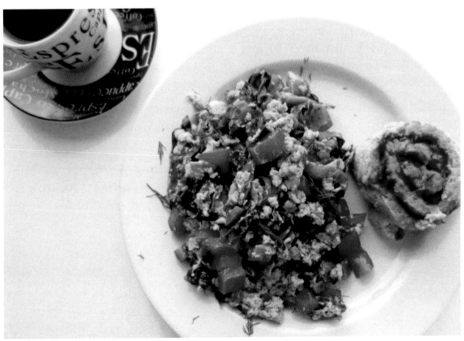

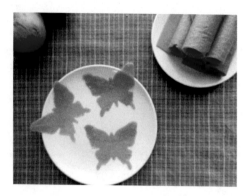

Dried Fruit Leather:

Ginger-Pear and Apple-Peach

Commercial fruit roll-ups often contain more corn syrup and chemical flavourings than fruit. The dried fruit snacks in this recipe make use of cooked and/or canned fruit and they're so easy to make. **Makes approximately 2 baking sheets**

Basic Apple-Peach

1½ c peeled, chopped peaches (approx. 2-3 peaches) or 1-15oz can peaches, drained*

1 apple, peeled and chopped or ¼ - ½ c applesauce

1 Tbsp lemon juice (to preserve colour)

2 Tbsp honey or sugar (optional)

Ginger Pear

5 pears, peeled and chopped or 2-15oz cans pears, drained*

½ tsp finely minced fresh ginger

⅛ tsp cinnamon

1 Tbsp lemon juice (to preserve colour)

2 Tbsp honey or sugar (optional)

Line a baking sheet with parchment paper and spray lightly with oil.

1. For both recipes: if using fresh fruit, bring all ingredients to a boil in a saucepot over medium-high heat. Reduce to a simmer and cook for approximately 20 minutes, until fruit is soft. Add water by the tablespoon if needed to prevent sticking. For both fresh and cooked fruit, move all ingredients to a blender or food processor and blend until smooth.

2. Pour over parchment paper-lined trays ¼-⅜" thick and bake in 135 – 170F oven for 4-6 hours, until fruit is no longer liquid or soft, and is pliable. Cut leather and parchment paper into strips and store in an airtight container, or cut into fun shapes with a cookie cutter.

Hint: Use almost any fruit and follow the basic recipe of 2 cups cooked fruit purée and 1 Tbsp lemon juice. Apples have natural pectin so adding applesauce to other fruits can help to make sturdy yet pliable leather.

* Use fruit canned in pear, pineapple or apple juice, not corn syrup or sugar. Reserve the liquid and use to mix into the smoothies in the *Breakfasts* chapter, serve with yogurt or add as a natural sweetener to the salad dressings in the *Salads & Dressings* chapter.

∞ Chapter 4: Breads & Baked Goods ∞

Bread, crackers, pizza... nobody wants to say goodbye to some of their favorite foods because of wheat allergies. The recipes in this section prove that it is possible to have all your favorite baked goods, and sometimes you can even slip some fruits and veggies into the mix.

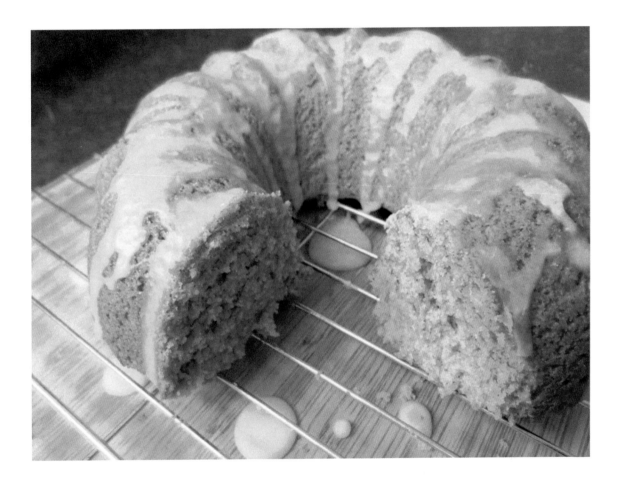

In this chapter:

Easy Wheat-Free Flatbread

Asparagus Flatbread

Olive Bread

Flax Meal Sandwich Bread

Cornmeal Bread (with Variations)

Sweet Potato Blueberry Muffins

Pizza Rolls

Chickpea Flatbread

Chocolate Beet Muffins and Cupcakes

Brown Rice Veggie Crackers

Sweet & Simple Dinner Rolls

Polish Blueberry Buns

Cantaloupe Coffee Cake

Easy Wheat-Free Flatbread

This quick, versatile flatbread can be used for anything from sandwiches to dipping to pizza crusts. If you like a thick, fluffy flatbread, spread all the dough on one cookie sheet. For a thinner style, divide it in two. Depending on your preferences and allergies, you can also add some extra herbs to the dough, like rosemary, onion flakes and garlic powder. **Makes 1 thick 9x13" flatbread or 2 thin flatbreads**

1 c sorghum or brown rice flour

½ c tapioca starch

1 Tbsp honey or sugar

½ tsp baking soda

1 Tbsp baking powder

1½ tsp corn-free xanthan gum

½ tsp. salt + more for sprinkling

¾ c water

1 tsp cider vinegar

2 Tbsp olive or coconut oil

2 eggs or 2 flaxseed eggs*

Optional

½ Tbsp dried onion

¼ tsp garlic powder

1 Tbsp dried rosemary

Preheat oven to 350F. Spray 1 or 2 baking sheets with oil and cover with parchment paper.

1. Sift dry ingredients in medium-sized bowl, adding in optional herbs if desired.

2. Mix wet ingredients together, add to dry ingredients and mix until smooth.

3. Spread the batter (or divide it for 2 thin flatbreads) over the parchment-covered pan with a wet spatula. Batter will be sticky; this is normal. Sprinkle with additional salt.

4. Bake for approximately 15 minutes until the bread is browned and feels springy to the touch.

* To make flax seed eggs, mix 2 Tbsp ground flaxseed/flaxseed meal with 6 Tbsp hot water. Mix well and let sit 5 minutes, until it is a thick gel. Cut xanthan gum back to ¾ tsp to avoid gumminess.

This bread freezes well and can be reheated in the microwave or oven.

Asparagus Flatbread

Delicious as a light meal or as an appetizer for a dinner party. Double the toppings to make two flatbreads instead of one.

Makes 1 thick or 2 thin 9x13" flatbread

One batch of *Easy Wheat-Free Flatbread* dough

6 asparagus shoots, cut diagonally into ¾" chunks

4 thin slices of red onion, cut into strips

Swiss or feta cheese as desired

Olive oil

Salt and pepper to taste

Preheat oven to 350F, spray 1 or 2 baking sheets with oil and cover with parchment paper.

1. Spread batter over the paper with a damp spatula and arrange asparagus and red onion over the batter. Add crumbled cheese as desired.

2. Drizzle or spray with a small amount of olive oil, and sprinkle with salt and pepper.

3. Bake for approximately 15 minutes, until crust is browned and springy to the touch. Remove from oven and cool.

This bread freezes well and can be reheated in the microwave or oven.

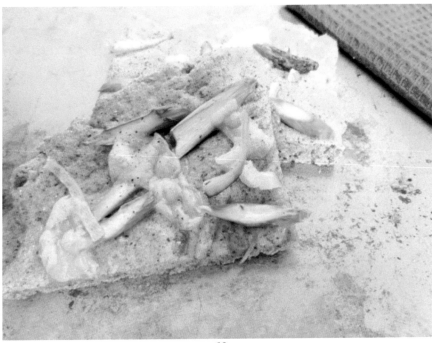

Olive Bread

Quick and easy, you can serve this to your friends and they'll never know its wheat-free. Serve as a side, a snack, or as an appetizer for dipping in olive oil and balsamic vinegar. **Makes 1 thick or 2 thin 9x13" flatbread**

1 batch *Easy Wheat-Free Flatbread* dough	1 tsp garlic powder
1 Tbsp dried rosemary	10-12 Kalamata olives, pitted and quartered
½ Tbsp dried onion flakes	Salt for sprinkling

Preheat oven to 350F, spray 1 or 2 baking sheets with oil and cover with parchment paper.

1. Fold rosemary, onion flakes and garlic powder into dough. With a damp spatula, spread over parchment paper. Arrange olive pieces over top and sprinkle with salt.

2. Bake for approximately 15 minutes, until crust is browned and springy to the touch. Remove from oven and cool.

This bread freezes well and can be reheated in the microwave or oven.

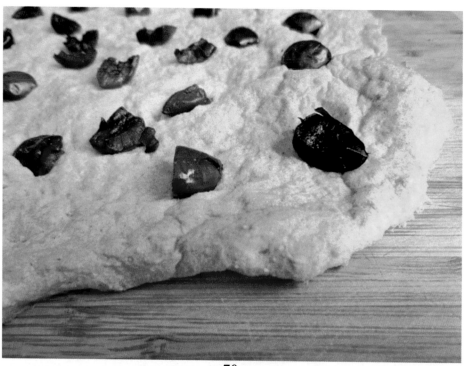

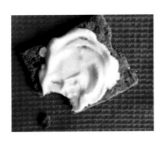

Flax Meal Sandwich Bread

One of the most popular recipes on my blog, this quick, nutritious flatbread makes a great sandwich bread thanks to its spongy, sturdy nature and short time to prepare. **Makes 1 9x13" flatbread**

1 c + 1Tbsp ground flax (flax meal)

½ c millet flour or brown rice flour

1 tsp salt, plus more for sprinkling

1 Tbsp baking powder

1 c water

Optional Seasonings:

2 tsp oregano

½ Tbsp dried onion

1 tsp garlic powder

½ Tbsp rosemary

Shredded cheese or parmesan

2-3 Tbsp raisins and 1 tsp cinnamon

2-3 Tbsp dried cranberries

Preheat oven to 450F. Spray a baking sheet with oil and cover with parchment paper.

1. Mix dry ingredients, optional seasonings and water together.

2. Let rest no longer than 5 minutes to thicken. Longer than this and the batter will become too thick to spread.

3. Spread flax batter over the sheet, about ¼" thick, sprinkle with more salt, and bake about 10 minutes, until firm but slightly springy.

This bread freezes well in slices and can be defrosted on the counter within an hour, or in 10 second increments in the microwave

Cornmeal Bread

With just a touch of sweetness, this versatile wheat-free cornbread can be served with breakfast, lunch, dinner, or as a snack. Optional additions, such as prepared salsa, zucchini or cheese make for healthy additions.

Makes 1-8" skillet or 8x8" baking pan

¾ c organic cornmeal	1 egg, beaten
1 c milk (cow, rice, or coconut, etc.)	¼ c honey or organic brown sugar
⅔ c brown rice flour or sorghum flour	¼ c olive or coconut oil
½ c tapioca starch	1 Tbsp butter or coconut oil
½ tsp xanthan gum	
2 tsp baking powder	Optional: ¼ c + 1 Tbsp salsa
½ tsp salt	1 c shredded zucchini
	1 c cheddar cheese

1. Mix the cornmeal and milk and let rest 15 minutes.

2. In a large bowl, mix dry ingredients together, from brown rice flour through to salt.

3. Beat together egg, honey and oil. Fold into dry ingredients with the corn meal and milk mixture. Beat until smooth.

4. Using the 1 Tbsp butter or coconut oil, grease an 8" cast iron skillet or 8" square baking dish. Pour batter into the dish and bake for approximately 45 minutes at 400F, until the top is crusty, and a knife inserted in the centre comes out clean. Allow to cool before cutting (texture will improve once cooled and set).

If using salsa, use ONLY ¾ c milk instead of 1 c and add salsa in with other wet ingredients. If using zucchini, salt the shredded zucchini and let sit in a colander for 10 minutes. Placing zucchini in a thin, clean dishtowel or cheesecloth, squeeze out as much water as possible and fold zucchini into dry ingredients before mixing in wet ingredients. If using cheese, fold into dry ingredients before wet ingredients.

Sweet Potato Blueberry Muffins

With three servings of fruits and vegetables, these muffins are delicious AND healthy. **Makes 12 muffins**

1 c sorghum flour

½ c millet flour

¼ c tapioca starch

1 tsp xanthan gum

2 tsp baking powder

1 tsp baking soda

2 Tbsp organic brown sugar

¼ tsp salt

2 eggs

1 c mashed, cooked sweet potato*

¼ c applesauce, puréed peaches or pears

3 Tbsp olive or coconut oil

1 tsp lemon juice

¾ c blueberries

Preheat oven to 350F. Grease a muffin tin or line with cupcake liners.

1. Sift flours together in a medium-sized bowl and combine.

2. In a large bowl, whisk eggs, mashed sweet potato, applesauce, oil and lemon juice until well blended. Beat in dry ingredients until mixed, then fold in blueberries. Scoop into muffin tins and bake approximately 25-30 minutes, until a toothpick inserted in the center comes out clean. Cool in the muffin tin 5 minutes, then move to a cooling rack.

* To make sweet potato purée, cut a large sweet potato into 3" chunks. Boil in a pot of water 10 minutes, until soft. Remove from water, peel and mash.

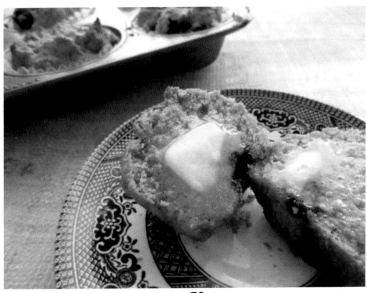

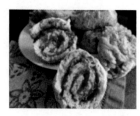

Pizza Rolls

Crusty on the outside and soft on the inside, these rolls make a great snack, dinner roll or even breakfast bun.

Makes 12-14 rolls

1½ c shredded zucchini + salt

1¼ c warm milk (cow, rice, or coconut, etc.)

1 Tbsp active dry yeast

1 tsp sugar

1 c tapioca starch

1½ c sorghum or brown rice flour + extra for dusting

1 Tbsp baking powder

1 tsp corn-free xanthan gum

1 tsp salt

1 Tbsp ground flax or chia seed mixed in 2 Tbsp hot water (or 1 egg)

¼ c olive or coconut oil

Pizza Sauce

1-6 oz can tomato paste

½ c + 1 Tbsp water

½ tsp EACH dried oregano & dried basil

¼ tsp cinnamon

1 Tbsp honey or brown sugar

¾ tsp garlic powder

½ tsp dried onion flakes

Salt and pepper to taste

Optional: ½ c shredded cheese + extra for topping

1. Salt zucchini and drain in a colander for 10-15 minutes. Wrap in clean kitchen towel or cheesecloth and squeeze tightly to remove as much water as possible.

2. Grease a baking sheet and line with parchment paper.

3. Mix together sauce ingredients.

4. Mix the milk, yeast and sugar together and set aside to rise, about 7 minutes.

5. Sift dry ingredients together. Add the flax mixture or egg, oil, and yeast mixture to dry ingredients and mix until a smooth batter is formed.

6. Generously dust a flat surface with rice flour. Turn the dough out on to it and dust with more rice flour. Knead 5 or 6 times to work in flour, so the dough is less sticky. Then dust again and, using a rolling pin, roll the dough out about ¼" thick.

Pizza Rolls, cont...

7. Spread a very thin layer of sauce over dough (extra sauce can be used for *Veggie Pizza*). Sprinkle with shredded zucchini and optional cheese. Very carefully, using a knife or spatula to help, lift the edge of the dough nearest to you up and over to roll the dough. Roll all the way to the opposite edge to create a large log. Using a wet, sharp knife, slice into rounds about 1- 1 ½" thick.

8. Lay the rolls out on the baking sheet, cut side up. Allow the rolls to rise in a warm place, about 30 minutes.

9. Top rolls with more shredded cheese, if desired. Heat oven to 375F and bake approximately 20 minutes, until slightly browned on top and a bit crusty on the sides.

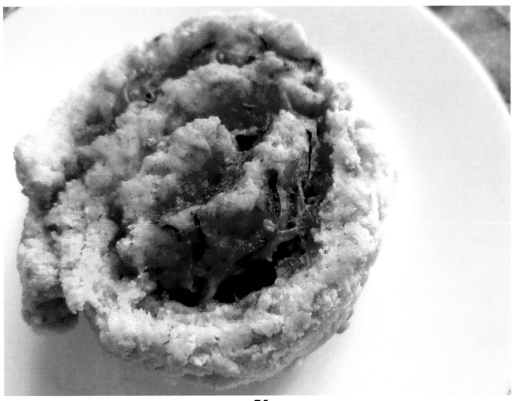

Chickpea Flatbread

Quick, customizable and delicious, this is one of my go-to bread recipes. It's also a wonderful way to scoop up sauces and dips. Chickpeas are a great source of protein.

Makes 6-8" flatbreads

1 c chickpea flour (a.k.a. garbanzo bean flour)	Optional: ¼ c boiled peas
¾ tsp baking soda	1-2 chopped green onions
½ tsp salt + more for sprinkling	2 Tbsp finely diced red pepper, sautéed 5-7 minutes
1 c water	Pinch of cumin
1 tsp apple cider vinegar	1 tsp caraway seeds
Oil for frying	Chopped fresh cilantro

Heat an 8" cast iron or non-stick skillet over medium heat. Add approximately 1 Tbsp oil.

1. Whisk together chickpea flour, baking soda, salt, water and apple cider vinegar until smooth. Fold in optional seasonings and vegetables.

2. Scoop approximately ¼ c batter into hot pan, spreading around pan. Sprinkle with extra salt and cover with a tight fitting lid. Cook 2-3 minutes, until bubbly on top. Remove lid, cook one more minute until edges begin to look dry. Spray or drizzle with a small amount of oil and flip. Cook 1-2 more minutes, until brown on both sides. Remove and repeat with remaining batter.

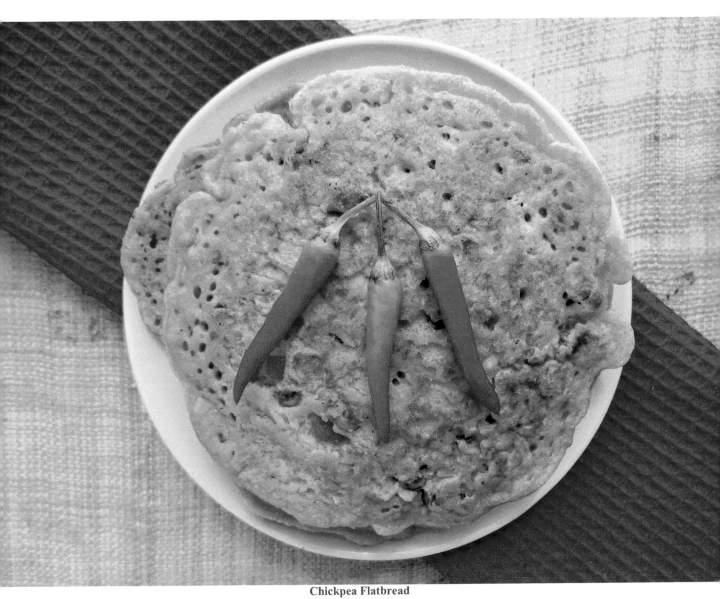

Chickpea Flatbread

Chocolate Beet Muffins and Cupcakes

Unusual, dark and earthy, you won't believe these are some of the healthiest muffins/cupcakes around. Even my husband, who won't eat beets, loves these muffins. **Makes about 12 cupcakes**

¾ c beet puree*

¼ c olive or coconut oil

½ c butter or dairy free alternative

½ c applesauce, puréed peaches or pears

1 egg

1 tsp vanilla

1 c sorghum flour

½ c brown rice flour

½ c tapioca starch

5 Tbsp cocoa

2 tsp baking powder

1 tsp xanthan or guar gum

Optional: ½ c chocolate chips

Frosting: 1 slice roasted beet

2 c icing sugar

2 Tbsp milk (cow, rice, coconut, etc.)

½ tsp vanilla

Preheat oven to 350F. Spray a muffin tin with oil or line with cupcake papers.

1. In a food processor, blend beets, oil, butter, applesauce, egg and vanilla until smooth.

2. Sift in flour, starch, cocoa and baking powder and pulse until blended. Fold in chocolate chips if using. Bake 25 minutes, until a toothpick inserted in the center comes out clean. Cool.

3. For cupcake frosting: beat together icing sugar, milk and vanilla until smooth. Fold in beet slice until frosting is pink. Remove beet slice and frost cupcakes.

*Approximately 1½ beets, baked roughly 1 hour in a 375F oven in a covered dish until soft, then peeled and puréed in a food processor.

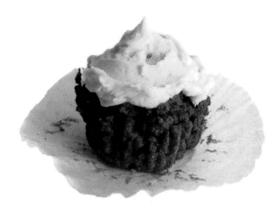

Brown Rice Veggie Crackers

As a kid I practically *lived* off vegetable crackers and wheat thins. Having to give them up cut my snack options in half. Eventually, I came up with this alternative for using up leftover rice, and found it healthier and tastier than any store bought cracker. I often double this recipe and make extra for snacking. **Makes 2 baking sheets**

½ c dry brown rice (makes about 2 cups cooked rice)	½ tsp dried garlic
1 c + 2 Tbsp water	2 tsp rosemary
½ Tbsp butter (optional)	1 tsp salt + extra for sprinkling on top
1 carrot, peeled	2 Tbsp olive or coconut oil
¼ red bell pepper	¼ c ground flax (flax meal)
¼ green bell pepper	¼ c millet or brown rice flour
3 grape tomatoes, or 2-3 slices tomato	1 Tbsp water
½ Tbsp dried onion	

Spray 2 baking sheets with oil and cover with parchment paper.

1. In a medium-sized pot swish rice under water. Drain the water and repeat 3-4 times until water runs clear. Add the 1 c and 2 Tbsp water and optional butter. Bring to a boil over high heat, reduce heat, cover and simmer for 30 minutes until water is absorbed and rice is soft.

2. Heat oven to 350F. In a food processor, blend cooked rice and all other ingredients together until a sticky mass is formed. Using a wet spatula, divide the batter onto the baking sheets and spread very thin, approximately ⅛" thick.

3. Using the edge of the spatula, score the batter by drawing gridlines about 1½" inches apart to create cracker shapes. Sprinkle with salt and bake 20-25 minutes until crackers brown, but not blacken (watch these carefully as they can burn quickly). Turn oven off, but leave crackers in the oven for another hour. As the oven cools, the crackers will harden.

These crackers keep well stored in a sealed container for up to 2 weeks.

Sweet & Simple Dinner Rolls

Light and fluffy, these dinner rolls will practically melt in your mouth. Note that the gluten free dough will seem sticky and too wet, but resist the urge to add extra flour. They'll turn out soft and with a tiny touch of sweetness. **Makes 10-12 rolls**

1 Tbsp active dry yeast

1 tsp sugar

1 c warm milk (cow, rice, or coconut, etc.)

¾ c sorghum flour

½ c tapioca starch

¼ c sweet rice flour/glutinous rice flour

1½ tsp xanthan gum

¾ tsp salt

½ Tbsp baking powder

1 egg or 1 flax egg*

2 Tbsp soft butter, olive or coconut oil

2 Tbsp organic brown sugar or honey

1 tsp apple cider vinegar

Optional: 1 beaten egg or 1 Tbsp melted butter for brushing on buns

Brush a muffin tin with melted butter or oil.

1. Prepare yeast mixture. Mix together yeast, sugar and milk and let rest *no more* than 7 minutes to bubble. Any longer time will result in over rising of buns, which will then sink.

2. Sift together dry ingredients. Mix together egg, butter, sugar or honey and apple cider vinegar and blend into dry ingredients along with yeast mixture. Blend until smooth.

3. Scoop batter into muffin tins, filling each one approximately ¾ full. In a warm place, let muffins rise 20 minutes.

4. Preheat oven to 375F. Brush optional egg or butter over buns and bake 13-17 minutes, until browned on top. Remove from heat and let cool in pans 15 minutes until set.

* To make flax egg, mix 1 Tbsp ground flax seeds with 3 Tbsp water. If using flax egg, cut xanthan gum back to ¾ tsp to avoid a gummy texture.

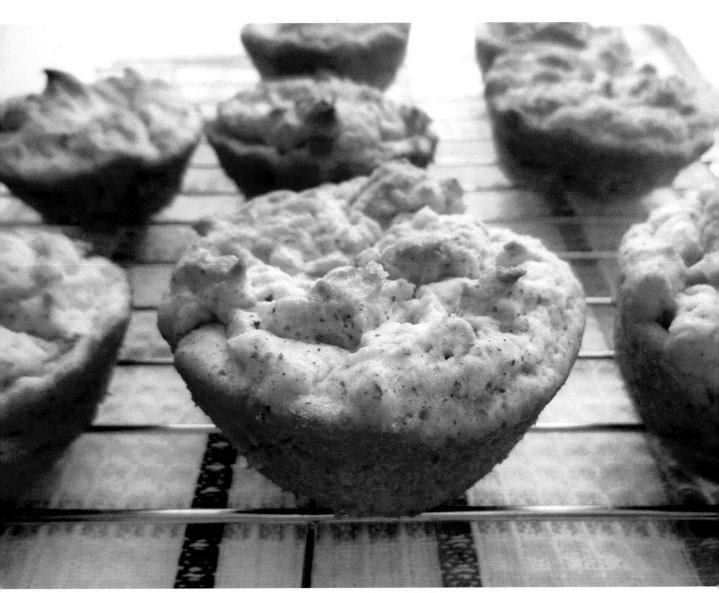

Sweet & Simple Dinner Rolls

Polish Blueberry Buns (Jagodzianki)

These buns pack a sweet surprise inside. This is a slightly "healthified" version of a traditional Polish bun, which can be modified depending on how sweet you like it. Serve for breakfast, afternoon tea or dessert. **Makes about 6 buns**

1 batch of *Sweet & Simple Dinner Roll* dough	Optional Toppings:
Zest of 1 lemon (optional)	1 egg beaten (for a browner, glossier top)
1 tsp vanilla	1 Tbsp butter, softened, crumbled with 1 Tbsp brown sugar
5-6 blueberries PER bun (approximately ¾ c blueberries total)	1 c powdered sugar mixed with 1 Tbsp lemon juice (as frosting)
¼ tsp sugar for sprinkling PER bun (optional)	

Brush a muffin tin with butter or oil.

1. Mix lemon zest and vanilla into the *Sweet & Simple Dinner Roll* dough.

2. Scoop spoonfuls of batter into muffin tin approximately ¼ full. Press 5-6 blueberries into the center of the batter. Sprinkle with sugar if desired. Scoop more batter over blueberries ¾ of the way up the tin. Repeat with remaining dough. Wet fingers and smooth over dough on tops of buns.

3. In a warm spot, let buns rise 20 minutes. Preheat oven to 375F and either brush buns with beaten egg or sprinkle with butter and brown sugar, if desired. Bake 13-17 minutes, until browned on top and firm yet spongy to the touch. Remove from oven and let cool 13-17 minutes in pan to set.

4. If desired, whisk powdered sugar and lemon juice together and drizzle over cooled buns.

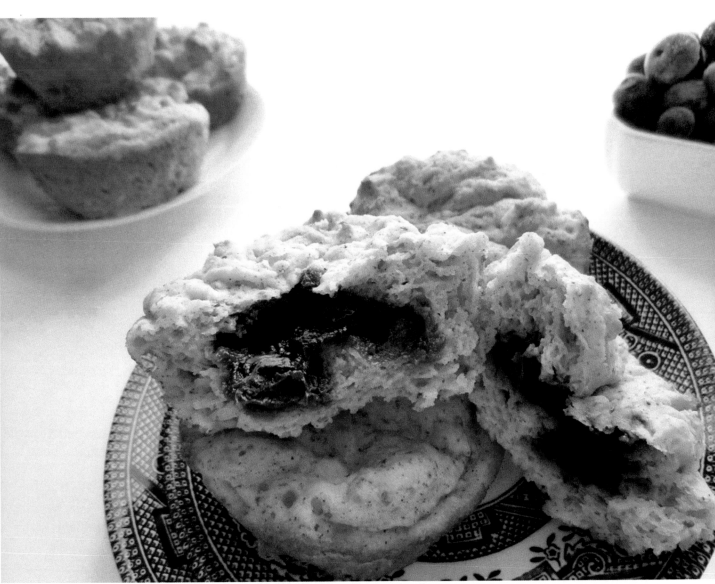

Polish Blueberry Buns, no toppings

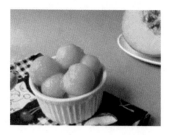

Cantaloupe Coffee Cake

This light cake has just a hint of cantaloupe and with puréed fruit, whole grain flours and half the sugar of most cakes, it makes a guilt-free breakfast cake or dessert. **Makes 1 6-cup Bundt cake or 1 9x9" baking dish**

2 c peeled, seeded and diced cantaloupe

½ c organic brown sugar

1 c sorghum flour

½ c brown rice flour

½ c tapioca starch

2 tsp baking powder

½ tsp salt

1 tsp cinnamon

½ c butter (or dairy free alternative), softened

¼ c coconut or olive oil

½ tsp vanilla extract

2 eggs

Glaze:

1 Tbsp cantaloupe purée

½ c powdered sugar

¼ tsp vanilla extract

Preheat oven to 375F, oil a 6-cup Bundt pan or a 9"x9" cake pan

1. In a small saucepan, cook cantaloupe over medium-low heat for 10 minutes, stirring occasionally until puréed and smooth. Remove from heat and cool. Divide as such: ¾ cups for cake, and 1 Tbsp for glaze.

2. Mix dry ingredients in a medium sized bowl.

3. In a large bowl beat together butter and cantaloupe. Add oil, vanilla, and eggs. Mix well.

4. Fold dry ingredients into wet. Pour batter into an oiled 6 cup Bundt pan or 9x9" baking dish and bake for 30 minutes, until top is browned and a toothpick inserted in the centre comes out clean. Turn cake over onto a cooling rack and cool.

To make the glaze:

Mix together the cantaloupe purée, vanilla and sugar. Drizzle over cooled cake.

❧ Chapter 5: Salads & Dressings ❧

For some people with OAS even fresh lettuce can cause a reaction. However, many greens can be steamed or cooked and served with wheat-free grains and baked vegetables to make great meal-sized salads. Kale in particular is a nutrient rich powerhouse that holds up well to cooking, boiling and baking.

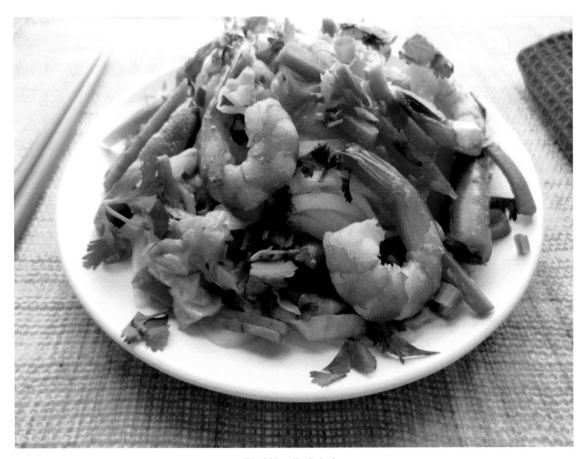

Thai Noodle Salad

In this chapter:

Wheat & Soy-Free Asian Ginger Dressing

Sweet Dijon Dressing

Blueberry Vinaigrette

Balsamic Pear Dressing

Thai Noodle Salad

Roasted Beet & Fennel Salad

Quinoa and Artichoke Salad

Peaches and Greens

Beet and Wilted Watercress Salad

Wheat & Soy-Free Asian Ginger Dressing

This mild, yet distinct Asian-style dressing works on everything from salad to stir fries and baked fish.

Makes approximately 1 cup

1 clove garlic, minced

1 tablespoon peeled and minced ginger root

¼ c olive oil

2 tbsp + 2 tsp rice vinegar

¼ c coconut aminos, gluten free Tamari or Bragg aminos*

1 Tbsp brown sugar or honey

¼ c warm water

In a large glass jar combine all ingredients, cover and shake well. You may need to heat the jar for 15 seconds or so to dissolve the sugar or honey, and reheat slightly before use.

Will keep in the fridge about 1½ week.

* **Coconut aminos** are a gluten, wheat and soy free alternative to soy sauce, available in health food stores, gluten free sections or online. If soy is not a problem for you, **Bragg amino acids** or **Tamari** are usually wheat free but not soy free alternatives that are easier to find and cheaper. Always check ingredient labels.

Sweet Dijon Dressing

Sweet and spicy, this dressing provides a sweet zing for salads or as a marinade for grilled vegetables.

Makes approximately ½ cup

2 Tbsp olive oil

2 Tbsp red wine vinegar

1 Tbsp Dijon mustard

3 Tbsp water

1½ Tbsp honey or sugar

In a small jar or container with a tight-fitting lid, add the dressing ingredients and shake the jar until well blended. If the flavour is too tangy, add more water and honey by the teaspoon to counteract the vinegar and mustard.

Will keep in the fridge about 2 weeks.

Blueberry Vinaigrette

Sweet and sour, and a fun way to get some fresh fruit in your diet, as blueberries are not commonly associated with OAS.

Makes approximately 1¼ cups

½ c blueberries (fresh or frozen)
4 Tbsp white vinegar
4 Tbsp olive oil
4 Tbsp maple syrup (or honey)
Salt and pepper to taste

In a blender or food processor, blend ingredients until smooth.

Will keep in the fridge about 1½ weeks.

Balsamic Pear Dressing

Another great way to add a touch of fruit and sweetness to a salad. Pair with a plate of steamed kale, wilted watercress, or mixed greens.

Makes approximately 1½ cups

1 15oz can pears in pear juice
½ Tbsp balsamic vinegar
2 Tbsp olive oil
¼ tsp sea salt
⅛ tsp pepper
½ Tbsp honey or brown sugar (optional)

In a blender, food processor or with a hand blender, blend all ingredients until smooth. Adjust seasonings to taste.

Will keep in the fridge about 1½ weeks.

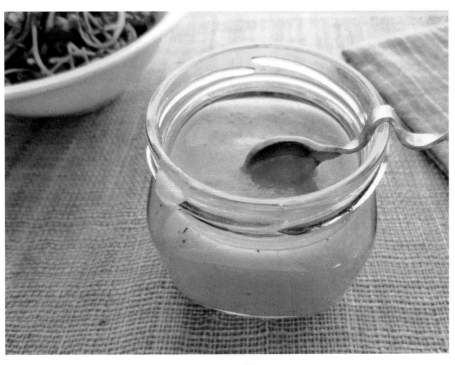

Thai Noodle Salad

I regularly make this salad for an easy dinner on a hot summer day. Serve in small appetizer portions or larger meal-sized ones. **Serves 2-4**

7 oz Pad Thai-style rice noodles, rice vermicelli or bean thread noodles

2 handfuls snow peas, washed and ends trimmed

1 Tbsp olive or coconut oil + more as needed

1" piece ginger, peeled and minced

1 clove garlic, minced

1 scallion, greens separated from white bulb and chopped

2 c shredded cabbage (red or green)

1 carrot, peeled and julienned or shredded

7 Tbsp *Wheat & Soy-Free Asian Ginger Dressing*

<u>Optional</u>: 12 prawns, 1 scrambled egg, ½ can organic corn, cashews, chopped cilantro or mint (if not allergic)

1. Bring a medium-sized pot of water to a boil. Add noodles and snow peas. Cook according to instructions on noodle package and snow peas are softened.

2. In the meantime, heat oil over medium heat in a large skillet. Add ginger, garlic and chopped white scallion bulb. Sauté 1 minute. Add cabbage and carrot. Sauté 10 minutes, until softened. If using prawns or egg, push vegetables aside, add more oil and cook prawns until pink, push aside prawns and cook egg until done. Add dressing and stir gently to distribute.

3. On a plate, arrange noodles with snow peas and place vegetables over top. Garnish with remaining chopped scallion and optional garnishes.

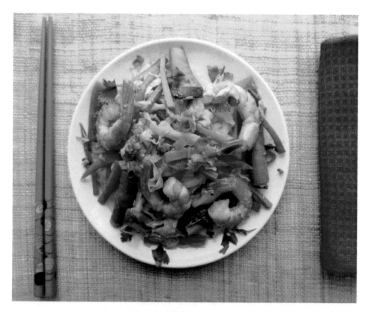

Roasted Beet & Fennel Salad

This salad makes a filling lunch or dinner salad, especially if served over a plate of cooked quinoa. Bake extra fennel and beets to keep in the fridge and make more salad throughout the week. **Serves 4**

1 fennel bulb, thinly sliced

1 carrot, peeled and cut into ½" chunks

2 medium-sized beets, scrubbed and stems/root trimmed to ½" long

1 Tbsp olive oil

1 tsp dried thyme

¼ tsp salt

4 c chopped kale or Swiss chard leaves, stems removed

1-2 Tbsp *Sweet Dijon Dressing* per salad

<u>Optional Toppings:</u> cashews, feta, goat cheese or bocconcini, fresh chopped dill

Preheat oven to 400F.

1. Gently toss fennel and carrots with olive oil, thyme and salt. Wrap in aluminum foil or oven proof dish with cover.

2. In another oven proof dish, bake beets, covered for 45 minutes, until soft. Add the fennel and carrots to the oven after 10 minutes and cook 30-35 minutes, until soft. Remove, cool, peel and slice beets.

3. Steam kale or Swiss chard in a steamer or metal colander over boiling water for 3-5 minutes, until wilted and soft.

4. Divide kale and vegetables. Arrange vegetables over kale and drizzle with *Sweet Dijon Dressing* and optional toppings.

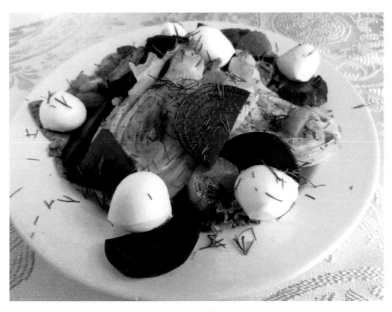

Quinoa and Artichoke Salad

Quinoa, kale and artichokes make for a nutritious, filling and protein packed salad that can easily be served as lunch or dinner. **Serves 2**

4 c kale leaves, stems removed, and roughly chopped

½ c quinoa

¾ c water or *Vegetable Stock*, or add ½ tsp cinnamon to water for extra flavour

½ 14oz can plain artichoke hearts, roughly chopped

1-2 Tbsp dried cranberries

2-3 Tbsp either *Sweet Dijon Dressing, Blueberry Vinaigrette* or *Balsamic Pear Dressing*

1. In a fine mesh strainer, rinse quinoa under cool water. In a medium-sized pot, bring water or stock to a boil, add quinoa and kale and bring back to a boil. Reduce heat to low, cover and simmer for 15 minutes. Remove from heat and let sit 5 minutes until water is absorbed.

2. Toss quinoa and kale with artichoke hearts, cranberries and dressing of choice.

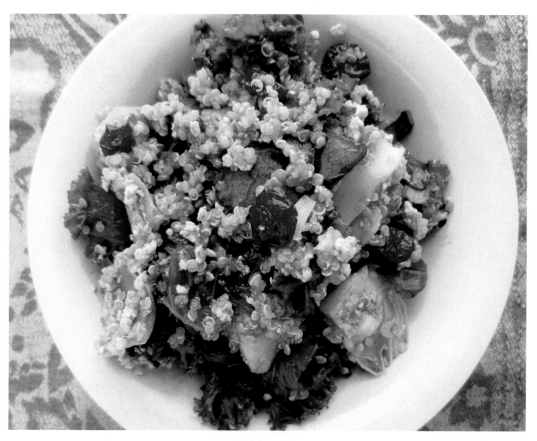

Peaches and Greens

Sweet and simple, peaches are a refreshing addition to a side salad. **Serves 2**

4 c loosely packed kale leaves, stems removed and roughly chopped

2 canned peaches, sliced (canned in pear or pineapple juice)*

3 Tbsp dried cranberries

4 Tbsp *Sweet Dijon Dressing, Blueberry Vinaigrette, or Balsamic Pear Dressing*

Optional: 2-4 Tbsp feta cheese, 4 Tbsp cashews

1. In a steamer or metal colander covered with a lid, steam kale over boiling water for 5-7 minutes, until wilted and bright green.

2. Divide kale and arrange over plates. Arrange peaches, cranberries and optional toppings over kale. Drizzle with dressing.

* Leftover pear or pineapple juice from canned peaches can be used to sweeten smoothies or to flavour yogurt.

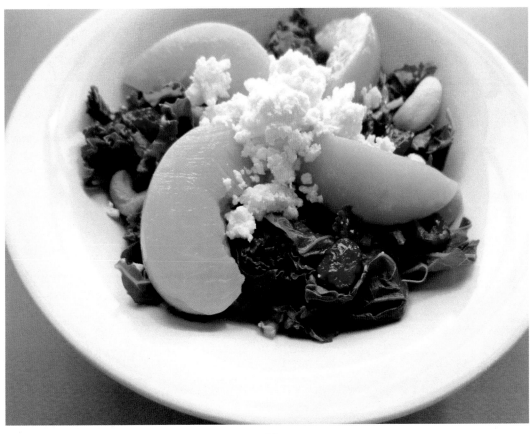

Beet and Wilted Watercress Salad

This simple side salad packs a sweet, nutty punch thanks to the beets and watercress.

Serves 2

1 bunch watercress, washed and chopped into 2" pieces	<u>Dressing:</u> *Blueberry Vinaigrette*
2 beets	OR:
<u>Optional:</u> Bocconcini cheese balls, feta cheese, cashews, grapes	1 Tbsp olive oil, ½ Tbsp balsamic vinegar, salt and pepper to taste

1. Bake beets in a 400F oven in a covered dish for 45 minutes - 1 hour, until soft. Remove, cool, peel and slice beets.

2. In a steamer or metal colander over a pot of boiling water, steam watercress for 2-3 minutes, until wilted.

3. Divide and arrange watercress in a plate or bowl. Arrange beets and optional cheese and drizzle with dressing.

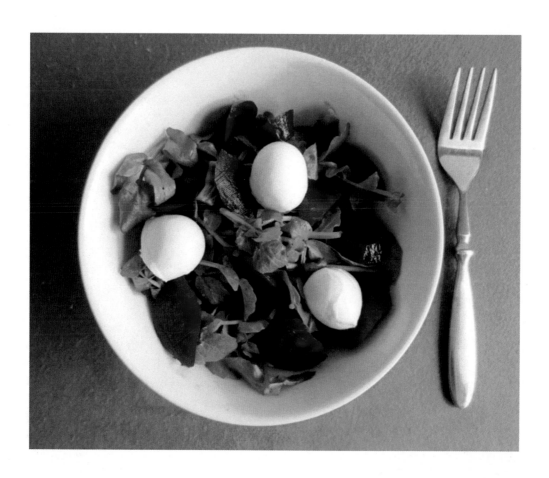

❧ Chapter 6: Soups & Sides ❧

Soups and hot side dishes are great ways to incorporate cooked veggies and even some fruit in to your diet. Soups with noodles and rice can make filling meals in their own right.

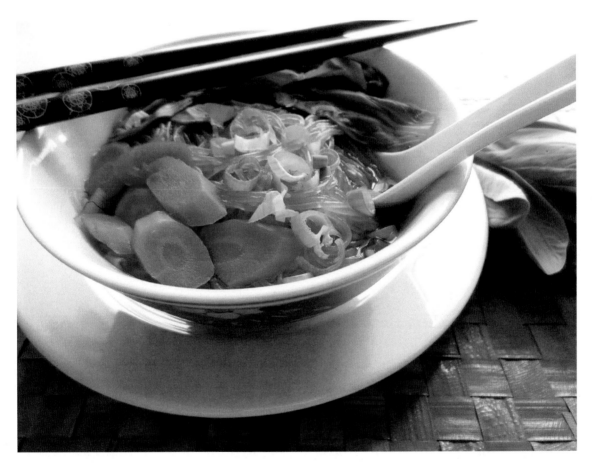

Green Top Asian Soup

In this chapter:

Vegetable Stock (and bouillon)

Store-bought stock can contain all kinds of hidden allergens, like wheat, soy, MSG, corn syrup, sugar and more. Making your own is simple and you can easily adapt it to suit your dietary restrictions. With two options to choose from, you don't ever have to be without a healthy stock at hand.

Vegetable Stock (makes 8 cups)
1 Tbsp olive or coconut oil
1 onion, peeled and quartered
4 cloves garlic, minced
2 carrots, peeled and diced into 1" chunks*
1 medium-sized fennel bulb, quartered*
4 stalks celery, roughly chopped*
1 bunch parsley, roughly chopped*
½ bunch cilantro, roughly chopped*
2 bay leaves
1 tsp salt
8 c water
*Or any combination of the above or other kitchen scraps equalling approximately 5 cups

Bouillon for quick stock (makes 3 cups)
1 medium onion, peeled
2 cloves garlic
½ lb carrots, peeled*
1 bunch parsley*
½ bunch cilantro*
1 medium-sized fennel bulb*
2 Roma tomatoes*
10 cremini mushrooms*
4 stalks celery*
½ c + 2 Tbsp salt
* Or any combination equalling approximately 6 cups, salt excluded

1. In a large pot, heat oil over medium heat. Add all ingredients up to bay leaves and cook over medium-high until softened, about 8-10 minutes, stirring frequently.

2. Add bay leaves, salt and water. Bring to a boil, then reduce to simmer for 30 minutes, uncovered. Strain and discard vegetables. Freeze in freezer-safe containers, or in ice cube trays. Once frozen, pop out and seal in freezer-safe containers or freezer bags.

1 ice cube = approximately 2 Tbsp

1. In the bowl of a food processor, blend all ingredients until a paste is formed, scraping down sides as needed.

2. Freeze in freezer-safe containers. The salt will prevent total freezing, making it easy to scoop out bouillon. To make a quick stock, add 1 Tbsp paste to 1 cup water, bring to a boil, then reduce heat and simmer 10 minutes. Strain if desired.

For a less salty option, reduce salt and freeze in smaller containers, such as ice cube trays. Once frozen, pop out and seal in freezer-safe containers or freezer bags.

1 ice cube = approximately 2 Tbsp

Green Top Asian Soup

This soup is so quick and easy, and can be served in smaller portions as an appetizer or in larger portions for a full meal. Almost any mixed greens can be used, such as bok choy, kale, Swiss chard, collard greens, beet greens or squash leaves. **Serves 4-6**

6 c *Vegetable Stock*

1 Tbsp minced ginger

1 carrot, peeled and thinly sliced on an angle

2 c bean thread or rice vermicelli noodles, broken or cut with kitchen shears into pieces about 1" long

1 Tbsp + 1tsp coconut aminos, gluten free Tamari or Bragg*

2-3 c greens of choice, washed and roughly chopped

1 Tbsp chopped green onion

Salt and pepper to taste

1. Bring stock, ginger, carrot and noodles to a boil in a large pot.

2. Reduce heat simmer for 7-8 minutes, until carrots and noodles are softened.

3. Add coconut aminos, greens and green onion. Simmer 2-6 minutes, until greens are soft (depending on greens being used).

4. Add salt and pepper to taste.

* **Coconut aminos** are a gluten, wheat and soy free alternative to soy sauce, available in health food stores, gluten free sections or online. If soy is not a problem for you, **Bragg amino acids** or **Tamari** are usually wheat free but not soy free alternatives that are easier to find and cheaper. Always check ingredient labels.

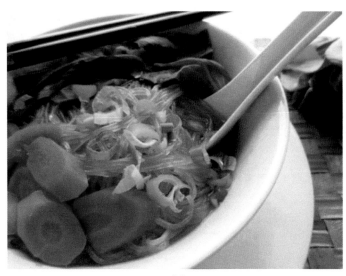

Tenerumi Noodle Soup

Tenerumi is the Italian word for the leaves and tender shoots of squash plants. While this recipe calls for squash leaves, kale leaves (without stems) or Swiss chard leaves and stems make excellent substitutes. This filling soup can easily be served as a meal in itself. **Makes 4 servings**

10-12 squash stems & leaves (approximately 4 cups)

2 large ripe tomatoes

½ lb baby potatoes, scrubbed with a vegetable brush and halved

1 carrot, peeled and diced

½ bunch parsley

8 oz gluten free brown rice elbow pasta

4 Tbsp olive oil

½ onion, diced

1 garlic clove, minced

Salt and pepper to taste

Parmesan cheese (optional)

1. Thoroughly wash squash leaves and chop into 1" pieces.

2. In a large pot, bring 3-4" of salted water to a boil. Plunge the tomatoes into the water and blanch for 2-3 minutes, until skins break and begin to peel. Remove into a bowl of cool water. Peel tomatoes and chop into chunks. Set aside.

3. To the pot of salted water, add the squash leaves and stems, potatoes, carrots, parsley, and pasta and bring water back to a boil. Reduce to a simmer and cover. Cook until al dente(approximately 15 minutes). Strain and reserve cooking liquid.

4. In a small pot, heat oil over medium-low heat. Sauté onion and garlic until onions are translucent. Add tomatoes and simmer until tomatoes break down. Add reserved liquid by the spoonful if needed to prevent sticking to pan.

5. Add tomato mixture to pasta and vegetables. Serve with reserved liquid to make a soupy broth.

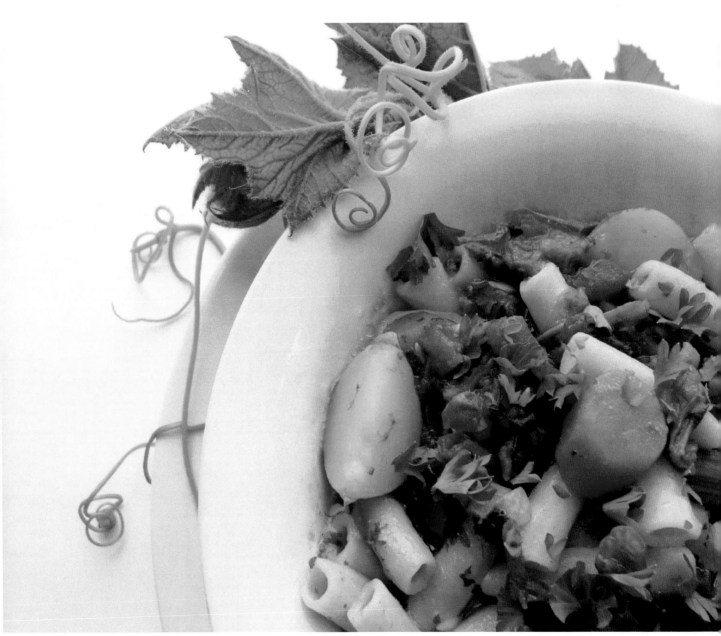

Tenerumi Noodle Soup

Watermelon Rind Soup

Surprisingly, watermelon rind is healthier than the inside pulp. Studies show that it is high in phyto-nutrients and anti-oxidants which are good for the heart and circulatory system and for building a healthy immune system.[108] Save the inner flesh for the cooked delight, *Watermelon Pudding (Page 132)*. The watermelon used for this photo was a small, sweet yellow watermelon, but any kind of watermelon will do. **Serves 2**

2 c chopped watermelon rind (directions below)	2 c *Vegetable Stock* or water
1 carrot, peeled and thinly sliced	2 Tbsp chopped fresh cilantro, mint or dill

1. Slice watermelon in half and, using a vegetable peeler or paring knife, thinly peel off the thick green outer skin. This part is inedible and can be discarded. Remove the inner flesh and reserve the yellow/white rind. Chop the rind into 1" chunks.

2. In a medium-sized pot, cook rind and carrot over medium heat for 10 minutes, until softened. Add water by the spoonful if needed to prevent sticking.

3. Add stock and herbs (or add herbs at end for a stronger flavour and if fresh herbs are tolerable). Bring to a boil, then reduce heat and simmer for 10 minutes. Serve warm or chilled.

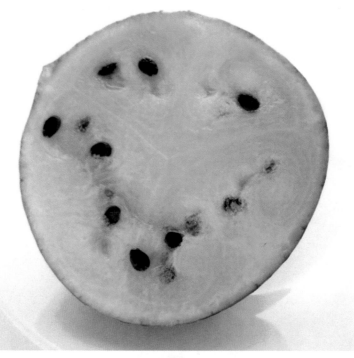

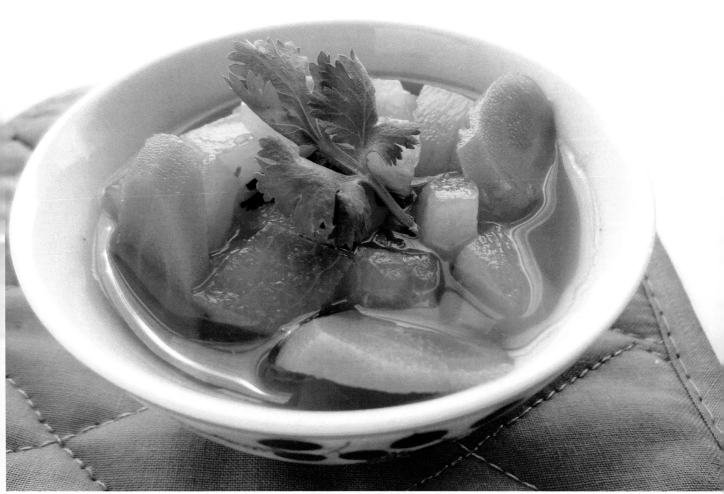

Watermelon Rind Soup

Hot or Cold Cucumber Soup

Raw cucumbers can be so refreshing, but allergies can cause some to miss out on them. By taking the extra step of sautéing, then simmering the cucumbers, it can be easier for most people to eat them. This soup is comforting served hot in the winter, and cooling if served chilled in the summer. **Serves 4**

2 c peeled, seeded and diced cucumber	1 c *Vegetable Stock*
Salt for sprinkling	½ c yogurt
1 clove garlic, finely chopped	1 Tbsp chopped mint
1 Tbsp coconut or olive oil	Salt and pepper to taste
2 tsp lemon juice	

1. Sprinkle some salt over the diced cucumber in a colander, leaving it to sit for 10 minutes to draw out moisture.

2. In a medium-sized sauce pan, heat oil over medium-low heat. Add garlic and sauté 1 minute.

3. Add lemon juice and diced cucumber. Cook on medium-high for 6-7 minutes, until cucumber is softened.

4. Add stock and bring to a boil, then turn down to simmer another 6-7 minutes.

5. Remove from heat and cool slightly. Add yogurt and mint. With an immersion blender, or in a blender, blend soup to desired consistency. Sprinkle with salt and pepper to taste and serve warm, or chill as desired.

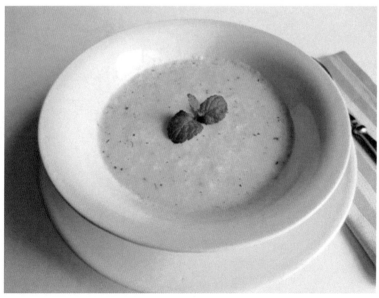

Coconut Cantaloupe Soup

Melons are often a forbidden fruit for people with OAS, but their sweet flavour is one to be missed. This Thai-inspired soup can be enjoyed warm or cold with the extra step of cooking the cantaloupe before blending the soup. **Serves 4**

4 c peeled, seeded and finely diced cantaloupe
1 Tbsp coconut or olive oil
1 Tbsp minced fresh ginger
2 Tbsp lime juice
1 14oz can coconut milk (1½ c yogurt may be substituted if coconut milk is not tolerated)

1 tsp dried lemon grass powder or 1Tbsp minced lemon grass
½ tsp salt
Optional Toppings:
Chopped shrimp
Chopped crab meat
Chopped mint

1. In a medium sized skillet, cook diced cantaloupe over medium-high heat until soft and almost entirely puréed, about 10 minutes. Remove and set aside.

2. In a medium sized pot, heat oil over medium heat. Add ginger and sauté 1 minute. Add lime juice, coconut milk, cantaloupe, lemon grass and salt. Cook 5 minutes until heated through. Remove from heat. If desired, blend in blender or with a hand-held blender to smooth any remaining chunks of cantaloupe.

3. Add optional toppings if desired.

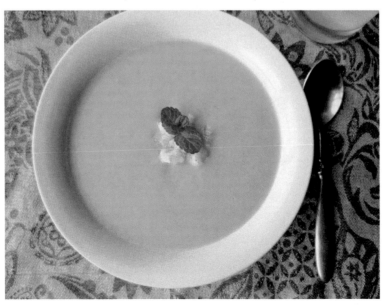

Mediterranean Roasted Peppers

Salty with a hint of sweetness, roasted peppers are a delicious side dish reminiscent of the Mediterranean seaside. Goes especially well with *Honey and Herb Root Vegetables* or *Quinoa and Artichoke Salad.*

Serves 4 as a side dish

12 mini bell peppers or 4 large red, orange or yellow bell peppers cut in halves or quarters lengthwise and de-seeded
1 large tomato, chopped into ½" cubes or roughly ½ c chopped cherry tomatoes
2 Tbsp olive oil

1 Tbsp fish sauce
1 Tbsp rosemary
½ tsp salt
1 clove garlic, finely minced

Optional: crushed cashews, feta cheese

Preheat oven to 350F and line a baking sheet with aluminum foil.

1. Lay out the bell peppers on the sheet with cut side up to create a small bowl.
2. Combine all remaining ingredients in a bowl and toss. Scoop small amounts of the ingredients into the pepper "bowls". Top with cashews or feta if desired.
3. Bake for 30 minutes, until the peppers are shrivelled and beginning to blacken.

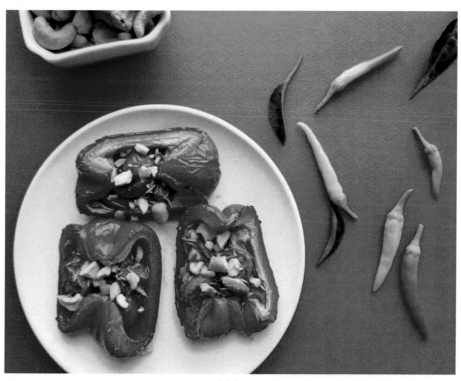

Honey and Herb Root Veggies

One evening while cooking dinner at my in-laws I used some of their potted rosemary and sage to season a bunch of root veggies. At dinner, my father in-law said "This is really good. Hey, you should put this in your cookbook." So here it is!

Serves 4 as a side dish

3 medium sized white turnips, peeled and cut into ½" cubes

2 medium sized carrots, peeled and cut into ½" cubes

OR roughly 4 cups of a combination of any of the following:

Sweet potatoes, carrots, fingerling or baby potatoes, turnips, or other root vegetables

1 Tbsp ginger, finely chopped

1 Tbsp fresh or ½ Tbsp. dried rosemary, finely chopped

1 Tbsp fresh or 1 tsp dried sage, finely chopped

1½ Tbsp honey or brown sugar

½ tsp salt

1 Tbsp olive oil

Preheat oven to 400F.

1. In an oven safe baking dish, toss all ingredients and bake for 35-40 minutes, until softened and browned. Remove from oven to toss halfway through.

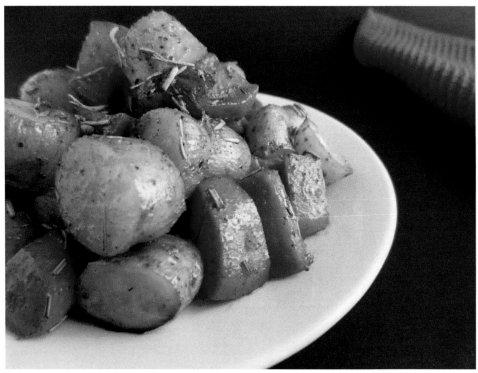

Thai Vegetable Wraps

A wonderfully simple, flavourful side dish that can easily be modified to become a meal. This is one of my husband's favorite snacks. **Makes 4 wraps**

1 egg, scrambled (optional)	1½ c shredded cabbage
1 Tbsp olive or coconut oil	2 c chopped kale leaves (stems removed)
1 clove garlic, minced	7 Tbsp *Wheat and Soy-Free Asian Ginger Dressing*
1 shallot, finely diced	
1 thumb-sized piece ginger, peeled and minced	4 rice paper wrappers (available in the Asian section of most markets)
1 carrot, peeled and grated	<u>Optional:</u> 4oz rice vermicelli noodles*

1. In a large skillet, cook the scrambled egg in the oil, omelette-style, until cooked on both sides. Remove from heat, cool and slice into thin strips.

2. In the same skillet over medium heat, add more oil if needed and sauté garlic, shallot and ginger 1 minute to release scent. Add carrot, cabbage, and dressing and sauté roughly 8 minutes, until softened. Add kale and sauté another 2 minutes, until kale is soft and bright green. Remove from heat and cool.

3. Soak rice paper wrappers in cool water 1-2 minutes to soften. Lay out on a flat surface and place 4 Tbsp of filling 1½" from bottom edge, leaving 1½" on both sides. Add ¼ of the egg strips. Lift bottom edge up and over filling, then wrap two sides over filling like an envelope. Roll forward to far edge.

* To make a meal out of these, cook rice vermicelli in boiling water 5 minutes, until soft. Drain and cool. Divide and layer vermicelli, then vegetables on a softened rice paper wrapper and wrap. With the rice vermicelli this can make 6-8 wraps

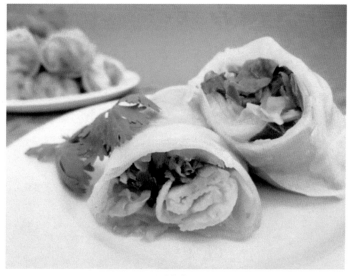

Sweet Potato Fries (3 Ways)

A healthier alternative to regular French fries for those allergic to white potatoes, baked sweet potatoes make a savory snack or side dish.

2 medium-sized sweet potatoes, scrubbed with a vegetable brush or peeled	Rosemary Fries: 1 Tbsp olive oil, 1 Tbsp chopped fresh rosemary, salt
Chili Fries: 1 Tbsp olive oil, ½ Tbsp chili powder, salt	Sweet Cinnamon Fries: 1 Tbsp olive oil, 1 Tbsp honey or brown sugar, 1 tsp cinnamon

1. Preheat oven to 450F. Line a baking sheet with parchment paper.

2. Slice sweet potatoes into French fry sized strips. In a large bowl, toss gently with any of the three toppings to coat. Arrange on baking sheet so fries do not touch. Bake for 15 minutes, remove from oven and turn fries over. Bake another 5-10 minutes, until browned. Remove from oven and serve.

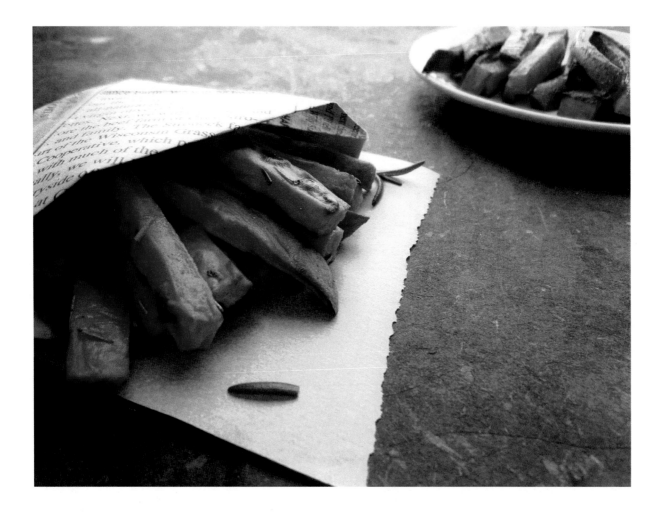

Sautéed Greens

Most greens can be sautéed and eaten. Bok choy, sui choy, squash leaves, Swiss chard, beet tops, kale, collard greens or mustard greens with a touch of carrot or fennel fronds all make great side dishes. Mix them up or grab a bunch from the fridge and pair them with your favorite main dish or a bowl of rice. Those allergic to lettuce may find this a good alternative to a raw side salad. **Serves 2**

1 Tbsp olive oil, coconut oil or butter	1 Tbsp lemon juice
1 clove garlic, minced	Approximately 4 c loosely packed greens

1. Heat oil or butter in a large skillet over medium heat. Add garlic and sauté 1 minute to release scent.
2. Add lemon juice and greens. Sauté 2-5 minutes until wilted (this will depend on the type of green used).

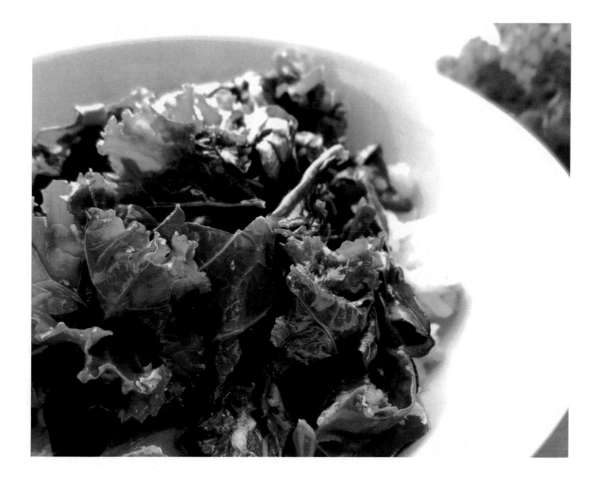

❧ Chapter 7: Mains ❦

While the soups and salads in the earlier chapters can make great meals in their own right, sometimes you just crave something a little heartier. These main courses can help you get that "full" feeling that many of us with allergies seem to constantly have.

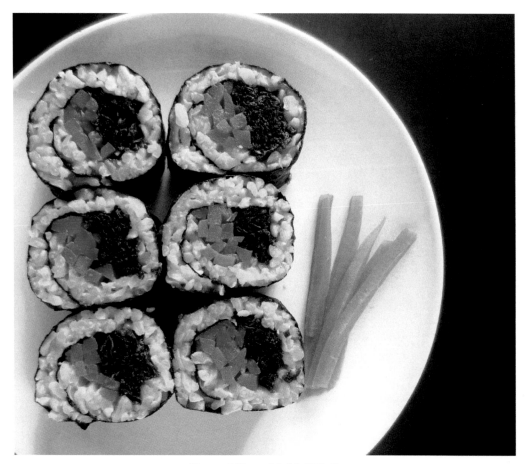

Steamed Vegetable Maki Rolls

In this chapter:

Asian Stir Fry

With its soy sauce, wheat, and nuts, Asian food is often out of reach for people with OAS. This recipe offers a basic brown sauce and variations that cater to all those allergies and makes a quick and satisfying meal. **Serves 4**

1 clove garlic, minced	<u>Sauce Ingredients:</u>
1" piece ginger, peeled and minced	2 Tbsp coconut aminos, gluten free Tamari or Bragg aminos*
2 Tbsp olive or coconut oil	1 Tbsp rice vinegar
1 c shredded green cabbage	1 Tbsp honey or brown sugar
2 carrots, thinly sliced	½ c *Vegetable Stock*
1 c broccoli florets	½ Tbsp tapioca starch or white rice flour
½ thinly sliced zucchini*	

1. In a large skillet, heat oil over low heat. Sauté garlic and ginger for 1 minute. Turn heat up to medium high; add vegetables and sauté 10-12 minutes, until soft. Add in prawns and egg, pushing the vegetables to edges of pan to create a space in the centre. Add extra oil if needed and cook until prawns change colour, flipping once. Add eggs, use a wooden spoon to scramble, then incorporate into the vegetables.

2. Whisk together sauce ingredients. Pour over vegetables and cook another 5 minutes, until sauce is thickened. Serve over brown rice, rice vermicelli, Pad Thai noodles, quinoa or millet.

* Alternatively, use any combination of the above ingredients or the following to equal 4 cups of vegetables: 1" slices asparagus, broccoli florets, green beans, ends trimmed and cut into 1" pieces, mushrooms, peas, shredded kale, spinach leaves, bok choy, sui choy, thinly sliced water chestnuts, or thinly sliced onion. Add softer leaves, like bok choy or spinach, after adding the sauce. Garnish with cilantro and chopped green onions if desired.

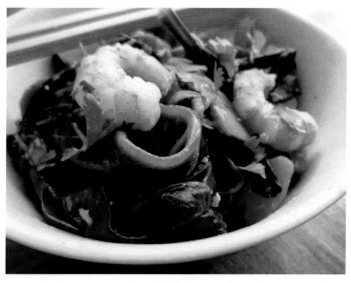

Vegetable Cabbage Rolls

A veggie version of my German grandmother's signature dish, *holopchi*, these vegetable cabbage rolls are packed full of healthy, vegetable goodness.

Makes approximately 30 rolls

1 c white rice	¾ tsp salt
½ medium zucchini, grated	½ tsp pepper
1 c grated cabbage	1-2 heads of cabbage
2 medium sized carrots, peeled and grated	Sauce
½ onion, chopped fine	2 c *Vegetable Stock*
1 tsp thyme	1-15oz can plain tomato paste
1 tsp oregano	2 Tbsp brown sugar
	1 Tbsp lemon juice

1. Prepare the head of cabbage one of two ways: freeze whole head of cabbage overnight and remove several hours before use to defrost. Use a sharp knife to cut core from the bottom of the cabbage head and gently peel off all the leaves. Alternatively, cut out the cabbage core and boil the whole head until the leaves are soft and start to fall off.

2. Mix rice, zucchini, carrots, shredded cabbage, thyme, oregano, salt and pepper in a large bowl.

3. Line a 9x13" casserole dish with extra cabbage leaves from the head of cabbage (optional, this is to help prevent the rolls from sticking to the bottom).

4. To roll cabbage leaves: cut out the bottom of the hard stem. Add 2 Tbsp filling to the bottom end of the leaf, leaving approximately 1" of leaf to the right and left. Folding the leaf like an envelope, lift the end of the leaf up and over the filling, then fold the right and left sides over. Continue rolling to the end of the leaf. Continue with the rest of the leaves to use all the filling. Place the cabbage rolls in the baking pan, tucking them in close together.

6. Mix together the sauce ingredients. Pour over the cabbage rolls to cover.

7. Cover the dish with lid or aluminum foil and bake at 350F for 1¾ hr-2 hrs, until rice inside the rolls is cooked through and leaves are soft. Baste with sauce partway through.

These freeze well. Defrost overnight in the fridge and reheat at 350F for 20 minutes.

Vegetarian / Vegan Lasagne

This vegetarian lasagne does away with the need for sourcing out wheat-free noodles and uses zucchini strips instead. Protein and veggie packed, this can easily be made vegan by omitting the cheese or using a vegan alternative. **Makes 1 9x9" baking pan**

1-2 large zucchini, cut lengthwise into 12 ¼" thick slices, approximately 9" long

Salt for sprinkling

1½ c *Vegetable Stock*

¾ c uncooked quinoa, rinsed and drained

½ c finely diced tomato

½ c finely chopped onion

1 tsp dried oregano

1 carrot, peeled and finely diced

1 c ricotta or cottage cheese (optional)

1 c shredded mozzarella or cheddar cheese (optional)

Tomato Sauce

Approximately 2 c chopped tomatoes or 1 15oz can tomato purée

1 clove garlic

1 tsp dried basil

1 tsp dried parsley

1 Tbsp honey or brown sugar

¼ tsp salt

¼ tsp pepper

1. Place zucchini on a clean dish towel or paper towels. Sprinkle both sides with salt to draw out moisture. Cover with towel and let sit while preparing remaining ingredients. Pat dry before using.

2. In a medium-sized pot, bring stock, quinoa, tomato, onion, oregano and carrot to a boil. Cover, reduce heat to simmer and cook for 20-25 minutes, until all liquid is absorbed. Remove from heat.

3. In a blender or food processor, blend tomatoes, garlic, basil, parsley, honey, salt and pepper until smooth.

4. Spread roughly ⅓ of the sauce over the bottom of a 9x9" baking pan. Lay 4 strips of zucchini over the sauce. Spoon ½ of the quinoa mix over zucchini, then top with another ⅓ of sauce. Lay out another 4 strips of zucchini, spoon remaining quinoa mix over strips, then spoon optional ricotta or cottage cheese over quinoa. Cover with remaining zucchini, remaining sauce, and optional shredded cheese.

5. Bake lasagne 30 minutes, or until zucchini is soft, sauce is bubbling and cheese is melted.

Veggie Pizza

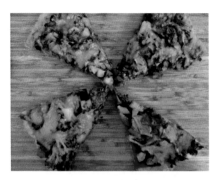

Who doesn't love pizza? Being allergic to wheat and vegetables doesn't mean you have to give up pizza. A wheat-free crust and sautéed vegetables makes for an extra-healthy, savory meal. The ingredients provided here are a basic guideline, so feel free to experiment. **Makes 1 veggie packed thick crust pizza or 2 thin crust pizzas with veggies divided between them.**

1 recipe *Easy Wheat-Free Flatbread* batter

2 Tbsp olive or coconut oil

½ green pepper, diced

½ red pepper, diced

¾ c broccoli florets

½ c diced zucchini

1 tsp dried oregano

1 c chopped kale leaves

1 c grated cheddar or mozzarella or dairy & soy free alternative

6-12 tomato slices

¼ c crushed pineapple

Pizza Sauce

1-6oz can tomato paste

6 oz water

½ tsp dried oregano

½ tsp dried basil

¼ tsp cinnamon

1 Tbsp honey or brown sugar

¾ tsp garlic powder

½ tsp dried onion flakes

Salt and pepper to taste

1. Oil one or two pizza pans and cut parchment paper to fit. Spread flatbread batter over parchment and bake in 350F oven for 12 minutes, until firm.

2. Mix together sauce ingredients and spread over pizzas (you may not require the entire amount of sauce, save leftovers for use in *Pizza Rolls*).

3. In a large skillet, heat the oil over medium heat. Sauté peppers, broccoli and zucchini for 7-8 minutes, until softened. Stir in oregano and arrange over crust. Arrange kale over vegetables.

4. Sprinkle with cheese. Top with tomato slices and crushed pineapple.

5. Bake in 350F oven for 10 minutes, until cheese is melted. Cut with a pizza cutter or sharp knife.

Fully Loaded Vegetable Pasta

Boiling gluten-free noodles and vegetables together makes for a quick and healthy meal. For those who can handle cooked tomatoes, there's a tomato sauce option. For those who want a one-pot, tomato-free version, skip the tomato and go straight to the stock! **Serves 2**

8oz brown rice pasta of choice

1 carrot, peeled and diced in ½" chunks

½ medium-sized zucchini, diced in ½" chunks

¼ c peas

1½ c torn kale, spinach or Swiss chard leaves, stems removed

Sauce

1 large tomato, blanched in boiling water and peeled*

1 Tbsp oil*

2 Tbsp finely diced onion*

1 clove garlic*

2 Tbsp red wine*

1 tsp fish sauce (optional)*

¼ c *Vegetable Stock*

1 tsp dried or 1 Tbsp fresh oregano

1 tsp dried or 1 Tbsp fresh basil

Salt and pepper to taste

Quick, tomato-free version: (omit ingredients with * next to them)

1. In a medium-sized pot, add enough salted water to cover pasta, carrot, zucchini and peas. Bring to a boil, reduce to a simmer and cook according to pasta package instructions, until al dente. In the last five minutes, add the kale or other leaves.

2. Drain, return to heat and add stock, oregano, basil and salt and pepper. Stir and cook 1-2 minutes, until noodles absorb liquid. Serve.

* Tomato sauce version:

1. Follow #1 above for quick, tomato-free version. While pasta is cooking, continue with the following steps.

2. Blanch the tomato in boiling water until the peel splits. Remove peel and roughly dice.

3. In a small saucepot heat oil over medium-low heat. Sauté onion 5 minutes, until translucent. Add garlic, sauté 1 minute. Add tomato and wine and simmer 10 minutes. Add fish sauce and stock. Simmer 5 minutes. Pour over drained pasta and toss with oregano, basil, salt and pepper.

Mango Vegetable Stir Fry

If ever there was a bright, cheery looking dish, this is it. This mango veggie stir fry makes me happy just looking at it, and even happier to eat it. **Serves 4**

1 c brown rice
2¼ c water or *Vegetable Stock*
2 Tbsp olive oil
1 clove garlic
1 Tbsp chopped ginger
½ c diced onion
1 tsp turmeric
½ each green & red bell peppers, diced
1 carrot, peeled and roughly chopped
½ zucchini, diced
½ c peas
1 mango, peeled, seeded and diced

1 tsp rice wine vinegar
1 Tbsp lime juice
1 c *Vegetable Stock*
½ Tbsp tapioca starch whisked into stock
1 Tbsp honey/brown sugar
1 Tbsp fish sauce (if desired, or use 1 Tbsp coconut aminos/or gluten free soy sauce and a pinch of salt)
Salt and pepper

Optional garnishes: cashews, chopped mint, dill

1. In a medium-sized pot, bring rice and water or stock to a boil. Reduce to a simmer and cover. Cook 30 minutes until water is absorbed. Fluff with a fork.

2. In a large pan, heat the olive oil over medium heat. Add the garlic, ginger and onion and sauté for 5-7 minutes, until onions are translucent. Lower heat to medium-low and add the turmeric. Sauté for 1 minute.

3. Add remaining vegetables and mango. Sauté 5 minutes, until softened slightly. Add all remaining ingredients and bring to a boil. Boil for 2 minutes, then reduce to a simmer for 20 minutes. Serve over rice with optional garnishes.

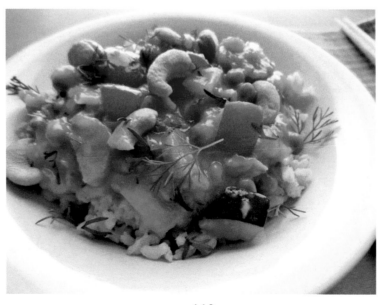

Black Bean Dip Dinner

Keep it simple, or dress it up with extra layers. This bean dip is versatile, and can be served with organic corn tortilla chips and vegetables for dipping, or over rice with sautéed vegetables. Make extra beans and freeze them for use in *Chocolate Chili* or more bean dip. **Serves 4-6**

1c dried black beans soaked in water overnight (or 1 15oz can refried beans)

2 Tbsp olive or coconut oil

1 clove garlic, minced

½ tsp cumin

½ tsp salt

1 tsp chili powder (optional)

¾ c prepared salsa

2 c kale, Swiss chard or spinach, stems removed and roughly chopped (or any type of green leafy vegetable that does not cause a reaction)

Optional Layers:

1 c yogurt/ sour cream, 1c shredded cheese, 1 c guacamole, 1c cooked brown rice

1. To prepare beans, soak 1 cup of dried black beans in water overnight. Drain and rinse. In a medium-sized pot, cover beans with 3 cups water and bring to a boil. Scoop off the brownish foam that arises. Reduce heat to simmer and cook beans 45 minutes-1hr, until soft, adding water if necessary to keep beans from scorching.

2. Remove beans from heat and drain. Heat oil in a large skillet and sauté garlic 1 minute. Add beans, cumin, salt, and chili powder. Using the back of a wooden spoon, roughly mash and stir. Remove from heat.

3. In a steamer or metal colander, steam kale, chard or spinach until bright green and soft. Alternatively, sauté the greens in 1 Tbsp oil over medium heat until wilted. Or, if raw greens do not cause an allergic reaction, use any greens of choice, chopped into bite-sized pieces.

4. In a pie plate or 9x9" baking dish, layer beans, salsa, and any additional layers. Top with greens and serve.

Steamed Vegetable Maki Rolls

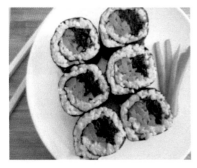

Although most sushi is raw (both fish and vegetables), these rolls call for well-steamed veggies, bringing out the sweetness of the carrots and making them safer to eat. **Makes 2 rolls, or 12-16 pieces**

1 c dry brown sushi rice or plain rice

2 ¼ c water

2 Tbsp rice vinegar

1 Tbsp coconut aminos, GF Tamari or Bragg aminos* plus extra for dipping

1 large carrot or small sweet potato, peeled and julienned in 1.5" matchsticks

4 kale leaves, stems removed

2 sheets Nori sushi (available in the Asian section of most markets)

1. In a pot, rinse the brown rice with cold water, swirl and strain. Repeat 2-3 times until the water is no longer cloudy. Add the 2¼ c water and 1 Tbsp coconut aminos to the rice. Bring water to a boil, then reduce to simmer for 30 minutes. Remove from heat, add 1 Tbsp rice vinegar and fluff with a fork. Cool.

2. In the meantime, steam the carrots or sweet potato in a steamer, covered with a lid, for 10 minutes, until bright and softened. Add the kale and steam another 2-3 minutes, until kale is wilted.

3. Lay a sushi mat on a flat surface (sushi mats are available in most Asian sections or markets). ***Hint*** Lay a sheet of waxed paper over the mat to keep mat clean. Lay a nori sheet on the sushi mat and scoop approximately ⅔ c of rice onto the mat. Carefully spread the rice out, patting and pressing it down. Leave 1" of bottom edge of nori free from rice.

   Divide the carrots and kale. Lay the carrots lengthwise on the bottom edge of the rice. Place the kale on top of the carrots. Following the directions on the nori sheet package, roll the nori sheet, pressing down gently at the end to seal with the sticky rice. Cut into 6-8 rounds. Repeat with remaining rice and vegetables.

* **Coconut aminos** are a gluten, wheat and soy free alternative to soy sauce, available in health food stores, gluten free sections or online. If soy is not a problem for you, **Bragg amino acids** or **Tamari** are usually wheat free but not soy free alternatives that are easier to find and cheaper. Always check ingredient labels.

Zucchini Boats and Quinoa

A tangy vegetable boat served alongside a plate of flavourful quinoa is a simple, yet tasty and filling meal. Quinoa's high nutrient and protein content makes it a healthy alternative to plain rice, especially for those with rice allergies. **Serves 4**

2 medium zucchinis	½ tsp dried oregano
½ red, yellow, orange or purple pepper, diced in small pieces	½ Tbsp each Dijon mustard, apple cider vinegar and water
16 cherry or grape tomatoes, cut in halves or quarters	1 c quinoa
1 clove garlic, finely minced	1½ c *Vegetable Stock* or water
2 Tbsp olive oil	<u>Optional:</u> feta cheese, cashews, grated cheddar cheese, rosemary

Preheat oven to 375F and lightly oil an ovenproof baking dish.

1. Wash zucchini, trim ends, slice lengthwise and scoop out soft centre. Finely dice the scooped out bits and toss in a bowl with peppers, tomatoes, garlic and olive oil.

2. Arrange zucchini halves in a baking dish. Divide the filling and pile it into the zucchini boats. Add optional toppings. Bake 30-40 minutes until zucchini is soft and a fork easily pierces the flesh. This will depend on the size and thickness of zucchini.

3. While zucchini is baking, prepare quinoa. Rinse quinoa several times and drain through a fine mesh strainer. In a medium-sized pot, bring quinoa and stock or water to a boil. Reduce heat, cover, and simmer for 15 minutes, until liquid is absorbed. Remove from heat and let sit, covered, for 5 minutes. Fluff with a fork and serve alongside zucchini boats.

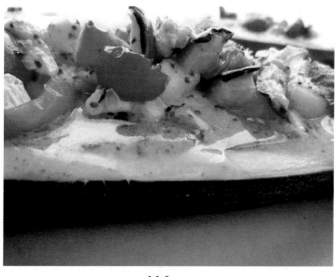

Chocolate Chili

The long cooking time of this chili helps to break down the allergen proteins in the beans and vegetables, making them safer for most with OAS to eat. The recipe is also very flexible so you can add veggies in or leave them out depending on what you have in the fridge and your own allergies. **Serves 6-8**

2 Tbsp olive or coconut oil	1 cup organic corn
1 small onion, finely chopped	2-15.5 ounce cans black or kidney beans (about 3 cups cooked beans)
2 cloves garlic, minced	
1 carrot, peeled and chopped	1-15 ounce can crushed tomatoes (about 2 cups chopped tomatoes)
½ green pepper, chopped	
½ red pepper, chopped	1½ tsp coconut aminos, gluten free Tamari or Bragg*
2 Tbsp ground cumin	1 Tbsp lemon or lime juice
1 Tbsp dried oregano	¼ cup dark chocolate, broken into pieces (about 1/3 of a bar of dark chocolate), chocolate chips or 3 Tbsp cocoa powder
1 tsp ground cinnamon	
½ tsp black pepper	
1 tsp salt	

1. In a large pot, heat the oil over medium heat. Add garlic and onions and sauté until onions are translucent, about 7 minutes.

2. Add carrot and peppers. Cover, and cook until softened, about 7 minutes.

3. Reduce heat to medium-low and add in cumin, oregano, cinnamon, pepper, and salt. Cook 3 minutes, stirring regularly to prevent burning of spices. Add some juice from the tomatoes, or a few chopped tomato bits, if needed to keep the spices and vegetables from burning.

4. Add the beans, tomatoes, Tamari and lemon or lime juice.

5. Turn heat up to a boil. Lower heat, cover pot, and simmer 15 minutes.

6. Stir in chocolate and adjust salt and pepper to taste.

* **Coconut aminos** are a gluten, wheat and soy free alternative to soy sauce, available in health food stores, gluten free sections or online. If soy is not a problem for you, **Bragg amino acids** or **Tamari** are usually wheat free but not soy free alternatives that are easier to find and cheaper. Always check ingredient labels.

Shroom-less Vegetable Pot Pie

Mushrooms don't agree with everyone, so this pot pie does away with them entirely while replacing the usual creamy gravy with a lighter one, making for a savoury and filling dinner that you can make all in one dish! It's also a great way to clean out the fridge of leftover bits and pieces. **Makes one 9" skillet or 8" pie plate**

1 batch *Pie Crust (Page 122)*	¼ c tapioca starch
2 Tbsp olive or coconut oil	1 clove garlic, minced
½ onion, finely diced	1 c *Vegetable Stock*
1 c diced broccoli florets*	1 c chopped fresh parsley
2 finely diced carrots*	1 tsp salt
½ c finely diced zucchini*	¼ c red lentils (optional)
¾ c finely diced russet or sweet potato*	** If a creamier gravy is preferred, use ½ c stock and ½ c milk of choice instead of 1 c stock
¼ shelled green peas*	
*Or a combination of any vegetables that equals about 4½ cups (i.e. shredded cabbage, fennel, cauliflower, corn, mushrooms, etc.)	

1. In a 9" skillet, heat oil over medium heat. Add onion, broccoli and carrot (or other firm vegetables being used) and sauté 7-10 minutes, until tender.

2. Stir in tapioca starch and garlic. Cook 1 minute. Add in zucchini, potatoes, peas, stock, parsley, salt and lentils. Cover and bring to boil, reduce heat to simmer 10 minutes. Remove from heat, and leave in skillet or transfer to pie plate, if using, and smooth surface.

3. Heat oven to 400F. Roll out pie dough about ⅛" thick. Cut to slightly larger than skillet or pie plate. Arrange pie dough over vegetables. Poke some holes in top of crust or slice a cross in centre for steam to escape.

4. Bake in oven for 35 minutes. Remove from heat and let stand 5 minutes before serving.

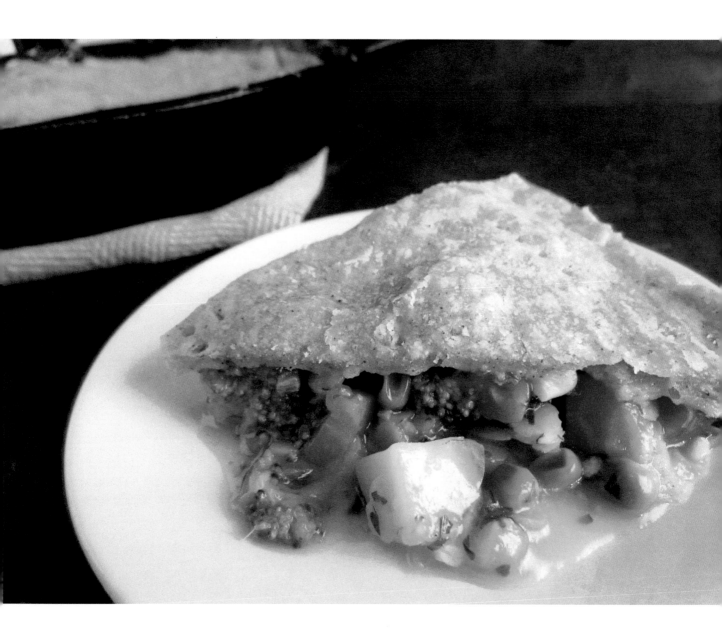

Fajita Bowl

A fun, easy, corn-free twist on the typical fajita, this fajita bowl allows you to customize based on your preferences and allergies. The long cooking time helps destroy allergen proteins so you can enjoy a giant bowl of veggies. **Serves 4**

½ onion, thinly sliced

½ each red and green bell pepper, thinly sliced

1 large carrot, peeled and julienned

½ zucchini, diced in ½" chunks

1 c shredded cabbage (purple or green)

1 c broccoli florets

2 Tbsp oil

OR any other combination of vegetables equalling approximately 4-5 cups

Fajita Seasoning

1 Tbsp white rice flour or tapioca starch

4 tsp chili powder

2 tsp salt

2 tsp paprika

2 tsp brown sugar

2 tsp onion powder

½ tsp garlic powder

½ tsp cumin

½ tsp black pepper

¼ tsp crushed red pepper flakes (or more if more heat is desired)

1. Mix together fajita seasoning in a sealed container. Unused mix can be saved for up to two months in a sealed container.

2. In a large skillet, heat oil over medium heat. Sauté onions until translucent. Add peppers, carrot, zucchini, cabbage and florets. Sauté 10 minutes, add 2-3 tablespoons seasoning and sauté another 2 minutes, until vegetables are soft and well coated. Add water by the tablespoon as needed to prevent sticking.

Remove from heat and serve over cooked rice or quinoa with steamed kale.

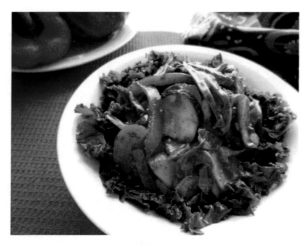

❧ Chapter 8: Desserts ❧

Although fresh fruit salads may be out of the question for most OAS'ers, there are still numerous ways to incorporate fruit into delicious desserts for healthy after-dinner treats. Cakes, popsicles and pies are all within reach.

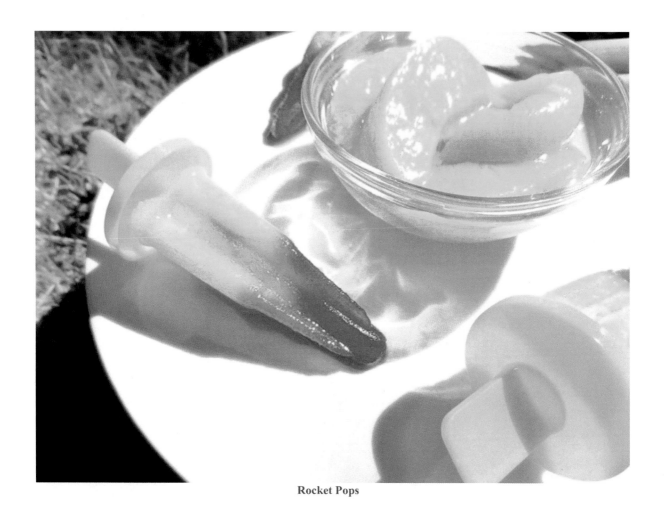

Rocket Pops

In this chapter:

Pie Crust

A quick, simple and versatile pie crust that can be used for *Fruit Pies*, *Schroom-less Vegetable Pot Pie,* or *Breakfast Peach Pie.* **Makes enough for 1 9" pie or 9 miniature hand pies**

¾ c either brown rice flour or sorghum flour	8 Tbsp butter or dairy free alternative, chilled and chopped into chunks
½ c tapioca starch (or arrowroot starch)	¼ c ice water + extra as needed
¼ c sweet rice flour	

1. Add all the dough ingredients except the water into the bowl of a food processor and pulse to blend, or combine in a bowl with a hand-held pastry blender or two knives, until blended and crumbly.

2. Slowly add the water and continue pulsing / or mixing with a wooden spoon until dough forms a ball. Add 1-2 tablespoons more water as needed and continue blending until dough is elastic but not sticky. Turn the ball of dough onto a sheet of waxed paper, wrap, and chill for 30 minutes before use. Let sit at room temp for 5-10 minutes before use. If it becomes too sticky after working with it, place back in fridge for another 5 minutes.

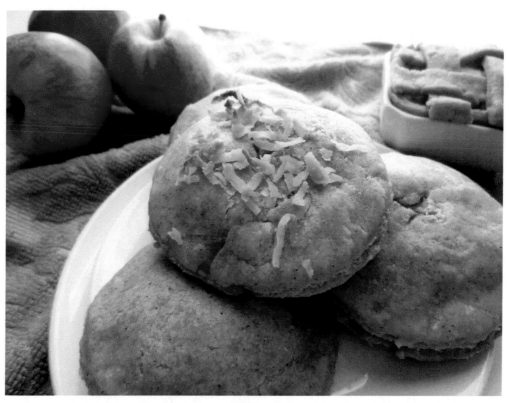

Chilled Pear Soup

So smooth you can drink it, this chilled pear soup uses canned pears to make a quick and easy appetizer or dessert soup. **Serves 3**

1-387mL can of pears in pear or pineapple juice

¼ tsp vanilla

¼ tsp dried ginger

¼ tsp salt

½ Tbsp honey (or other sweetener)

5 Tbsp water

1. Blend all ingredients together in a blender or food processor. Chill and serve.

Alternatively, use 2 fresh pears, peeled and diced. Cook over medium-high heat for 15-20 minutes with ¼ c water. Once pears have cooked down, add remaining ingredients and blend. Serve warm or chilled.

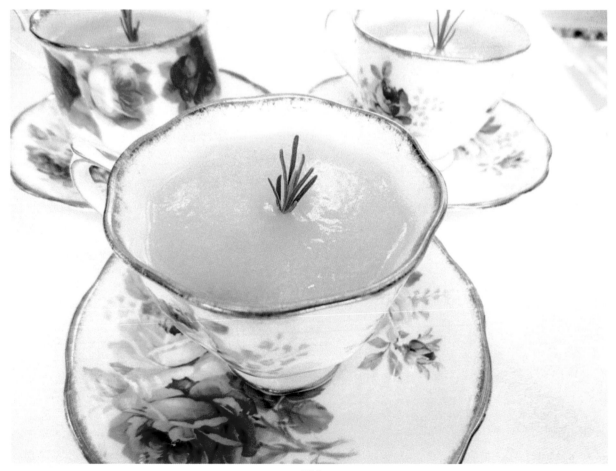

Spiced Chocolate Applesauce Cake

A fluffy cake that is naturally sweet with a delicate applesauce and cocoa flavour, no one will ever know it's actually wheat free and good for you.

Makes one 9x13" cake or one 12 cup bundt pan

2 Tbsp brown sugar, honey or maple syrup	¼ c cocoa
¼ c olive oil, coconut oil or soft butter	¾ c tapioca starch
2 eggs	1 tsp cinnamon
1 ⅓ c applesauce, puréed peaches or pears	½ tsp cloves
1 Tbsp apple cider vinegar	2 tsp baking powder
1 tsp vanilla	1 tsp baking soda
1 c sorghum flour	1½ tsp xanthan gum
¼ c millet flour	
	Optional: ¾ c chocolate chips

Grease a 9x13" baking pan or 12 cup bundt pan. Preheat oven to 350.

1. Using an electric mixer, beat the sugar, oil, and eggs until fluffy. Add the applesauce, cider vinegar and vanilla. Beat 1-2 minutes.

2. In a separate bowl, mix together all the dry ingredients. Slowly fold dry ingredients into the applesauce and egg mixture. Fold in chocolate chips if using.

3. Pour batter into pan and bake for 35-40 minutes or until a toothpick inserted into the middle comes out clean.

4. Sprinkle with a bit of powdered sugar if desired.

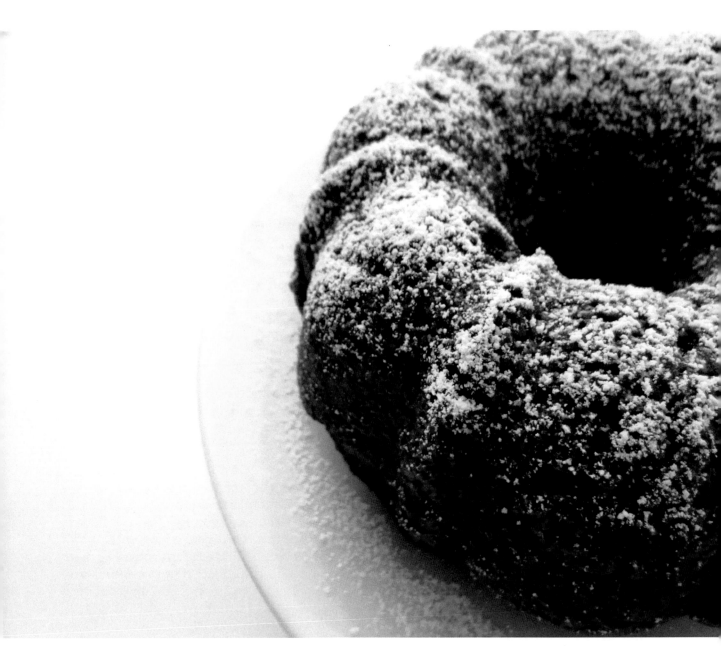

Spiced Chocolate Applesauce Cake

Mini Fruit Pie

Use any combination of fruit that works for you, apples, pears, peaches, blueberries, blackberries or mangos, just follow the basic recipe and enjoy. **Makes 9 small hand pies or 5-6 ramekins**

1 batch *Pie Crust (Page 122)*	¾ tsp vanilla
2 c peeled, de-seeded and finely diced apples (about 2 apples)	¼ tsp salt
¼ tsp cinnamon	Optional: 1 Tbsp brown sugar for filling, 1 Tbsp brown sugar and ¼ tsp cinnamon for sprinkling on top, flaked coconut for topping
1 tsp lemon juice	
1 Tbsp rice flour + extra for sprinkling	

Preheat oven to 350F, oil a baking sheet and cover with parchment paper.

1. In a saucepot over medium-high heat, heat sliced apples, lemon juice, rice flour and optional sugar. Cook roughly 10 minutes, until apples are soft and sticky. Add water by the tablespoon as necessary to prevent sticking to pot.

2. Remove from heat and stir in vanilla and salt.

3. Roll out the dough about ⅛" thick on a flat surface sprinkled with rice flour and a floured rolling pin, or between two sheets of waxed paper. If dough is too hard, let rest at room temperature 5-10 minutes before use.

4. **To make individual ramekin pies:** Grease ramekins and arrange pieces of dough in the bottom of ramekins, with just ⅛" hanging over edge. Add filling, until ½" below rim. Slice strips of dough roughly ¾" wide and length of ramekin. Arrange over filled ramekins in a latticework style. Pinch top together with bottom crust. Place on baking sheet and bake 20 minutes, until dough is firm but flexible.

   To make individual hand pies: Using a circular object of the desired size (i.e. a glass with a large rim, the edge of a glass jar, or a metal jar lid) cut out circles to make the tops and bottoms of the pies and arrange on baking sheet. Fill with approximately 2 Tbsp filling, leaving ¼" around edges. Dampen edges with a wet finger, cover with another piece and pinch edges to seal. Using a fork or knife, poke holes in the top to let steam escape. Arrange on baking sheet. Keep rerolling and cutting out the dough as needed. If dough becomes too sticky, pop back in the fridge 5-10 minutes. Top with optional toppings. Bake 15 minutes, until dough is firm but flexible.

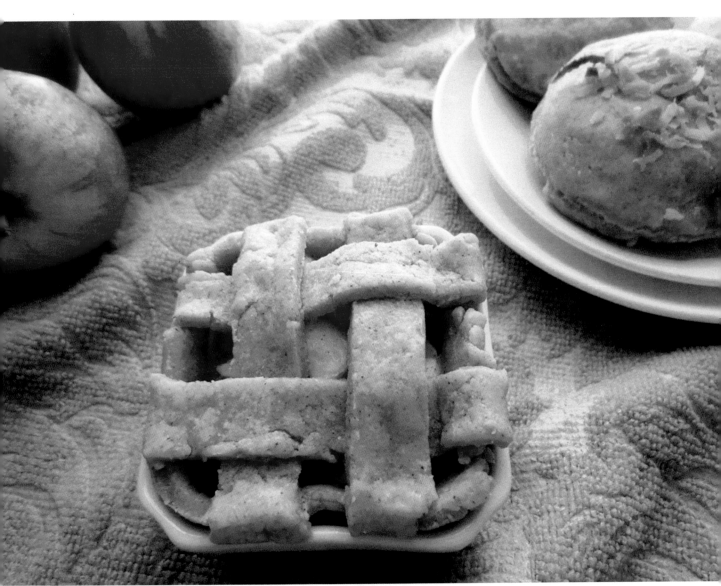

Mini Fruit Pies

Blueberry Crisp

Fruit crisp is so simple to make, and this blueberry one is a classic favorite for potlucks and family dinners. Double it to take to parties and share with friends. **Makes 1 - 9x9" baking dish.**

3 c washed blueberries (fresh or frozen)	½ c brown rice flour
1 Tbsp white rice flour	¼ tsp salt
1 tsp cinnamon	¼ c butter
⅛ tsp salt	¼ c brown sugar
1 Tbsp water	½ tsp vanilla
	¼ tsp cinnamon

Preheat oven to 375F. Lightly oil a 9x9" baking dish, or several ramekins.

1. Gently mix blueberries, rice flour, cinnamon, salt and water together. Spread in baking dish.

2. With a pastry blender or fingers, crumble together rice flour, salt, butter, sugar, vanilla, and cinnamon. Sprinkle over the blueberries and bake for 35 minutes.

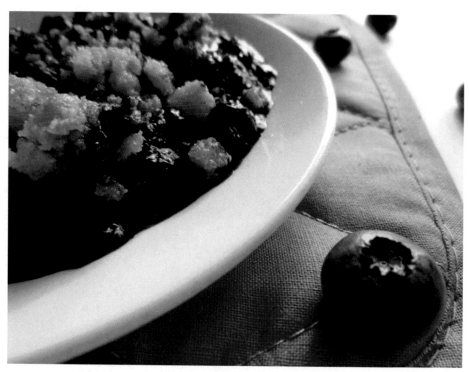

Blueberry Polenta Cake

Dense and moist, this polenta cake sneaks in applesauce for a hint of sweetness and an extra serving of fruit. Serve for dessert or afternoon tea. **Makes 1 6½" skillet or 1 9x9" baking dish**

¾ c sorghum flour	1 egg
¾ c organic cornmeal	⅓ c yogurt
¼ c tapioca	2 Tbsp lemon juice
1 tsp baking powder	¼ tsp grated lemon rind
¼ tsp salt	¾ c blueberries
½ c brown sugar	<u>Glaze (optional)</u>
¼ c olive oil, coconut oil, or butter	3 Tbsp lemon juice
¼ c applesauce or puréed peaches	1 c powdered sugar

Preheat oven to 350F. Grease a 6 ½" cast iron skillet or 9x9" cake pan.

1. Sift together the dry ingredients. In a large bowl, whisk together the oil, applesauce, egg, yogurt, lemon juice and rind. Beat in the dry ingredients. Fold in blueberries.

2. Bake in preheated oven for 35 minutes, until a toothpick inserted in the centre comes out clean. Cool on rack.

3. Whisk together lemon juice and sugar glaze. Insert toothpick into cake at intervals and pour glaze over the cake.

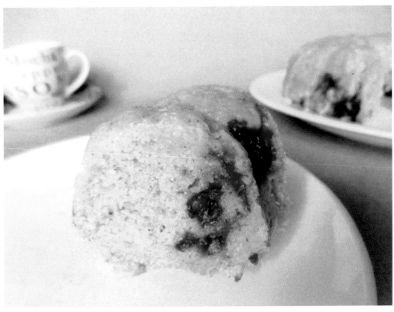

Rocket Pops

A great combo of fresh and canned fruit that makes eating fruit fun. Layer the three mixes to create a fiery effect!

Serves 4-6

¾ c pomegranate juice

¾ c canned, puréed peaches

¾ c canned applesauce or puréed pears

1. Mix two tablespoons of the applesauce with the pomegranate juice to thicken the pomegranate juice. Divide the pomegranate-applesauce mix between popsicle molds.

2. Divide and scoop the puréed peaches over the pomegranate-applesauce mix.

3. Divide and scoop the applesauce over the peach purée. Add sticks and freeze for several hours until frozen solid.

Purple Popsicles

These popsicles are a great way to make use of two fruits not commonly related to OAS.

Serves 4-6

1 c pomegranate juice

1 ½ c blueberries (fresh or frozen)

2 Tbsp honey (or sugar or alternative sweetener)

1. In a blender, purée the blueberries with the pomegranate and honey until smooth. Pour into popsicle molds, add sticks and freeze for several hours, until frozen solid.

To remove from molds, pour warm water over the molds and wiggle the sticks until the popsicles come free.

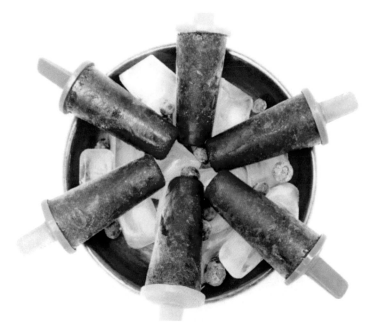

Chocolate Orange Pudding

This microwaved pudding is so quick and easy to make you'll never need to buy pre-packaged pudding again. Alternatively, this can be heated on the stove rather than microwaved. **Serves 4**

3 Tbsp cocoa

4 Tbsp tapioca or corn starch

½ tsp salt

2.5 Tbsp sugar, honey or stevia equivalent

2 c milk (cow, rice, or coconut, etc.)

4 oz orange flavoured dark chocolate, chopped (i.e. one bar of dark chocolate)

1 tsp vanilla

1. In a microwave safe bowl, whisk together the cocoa, starch and salt. Whisk in the milk a little bit at a time to avoid clumps. Whisk in the sugar, honey or stevia. Add the chopped dark chocolate.

2. Microwave the pudding for 2 minutes on high, stir, then cook in 30 second increments, stirring and heating until chocolate is melted and pudding becomes shiny and thick. Add in the vanilla.

3. Divide the pudding into serving cups and chill until cool and thick.

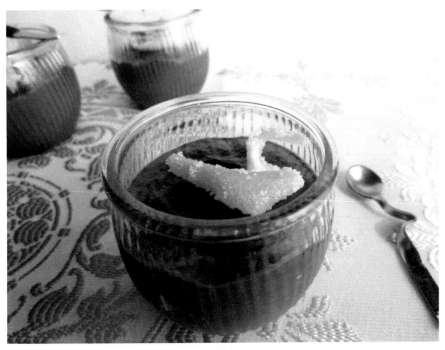

Watermelon Pudding

A traditional Sicilian desert, this is a fun way to eat cooked watermelon. Depending on your tastes, you may choose to do without the vanilla and cinnamon to enhance the sweet, simple watermelon flavour. Save the rind to make *Watermelon Rind Soup.*
Makes approximately 2 cups of pudding

2 c watermelon purée (about 2.5 - 3 cups cubed melon)

2 Tbsp water

¼ c tapioca starch

¼ tsp cinnamon (optional)

¼ c brown sugar or honey

½ tsp vanilla (optional)

Optional garnishes: chocolate shavings, whipped cream, pistachios, chocolate chips

1. Peel and de-seed watermelon, then cut into small chunks. In a blender, food processor, or using a hand blender, blend watermelon until smooth. Strain through a fine mesh strainer, flour sac or cheesecloth.

2. Whisk 2 Tbsp water with the tapioca starch and cinnamon until smooth. Set aside.

3. In a medium-sized pot, heat the watermelon purée over medium-high heat. Bring watermelon to a boil and whisk in honey. Cook for 10 minutes. Whisk in the tapioca-water mix, reduce heat to simmer, and stir constantly until thickened, about 8 minutes.

4. Remove from heat, whisk in vanilla and pour into serving cups. Chill 2 hours before serving with optional garnishes.

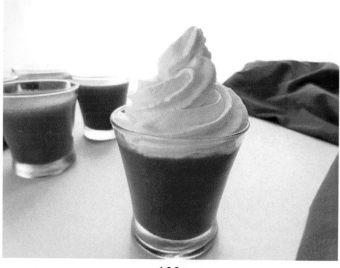

REFERENCES

[1] Skypala IJ, Calderon MA, Leeds AR, Emery P, Till SJ, Durham SR. "Development and validation of a structured questionnaire for the diagnosis of oral allergy syndrome in subjects with seasonal allergic rhinitis during the UK birch pollen season," *Clinical and Experimental Allergy: Journal of the British Society for Allergy and Clinical Immunolog,* July 2011, 41 (7).

[2] Various studies throughout Europe have produced differing numbers on the exact percentage of OAS sufferers, but all appear to agree that OAS is the leading cause of food allergies. Variations in percentage may also be based on a number of factors, including different methods for testing and varying numbers and locations of subjects.
For example, one Italian study (Asero1) suggested that oral allergy syndrome was the leading cause of allergies in Italy, causing 55% of food allergies. However, Skypala (2011) suggests OAS is the cause of approximately 60% of food allergies, and another (Roehr) puts the number much higher, at 66.6%.

For Italy, see R. Asero1, L. Antonicelli, A. Arena, L. Bommarito, B. Caruso, M. Crivellaro, M. De Carli, E. Della Torre, F. Della Torre, E. Heffler, F. Lodi Rizzini, R. Longo, G. Manzotti, M. Marcotulli, A. Melchiorre, P. Minale, P. Morandi, B. Moreni, A. Moschella, F. Murzilli, F. Nebiolo, M. Poppa, S. Randazzo, G. Rossi, G. E. Senna, "EpidemAAITO: Features of food allergy in Italian adults attending allergy clinics: a multi-centre study," *Clinical & Experimental Allergy,* Volume 39, Issue 4, April 2009, 547–555.

A study of residents of Berlin, Germany puts the number much higher, at 66.6%. See C. C. Roehr, G. Edenharterw, S. Reimannz, I. Ehlersz, M. Wormz, T. Zuberbierz and B. Niggemann, "Food allergy and non-allergic food hypersensitivity in children and adolescents," *Clinical & Experimental Allergy,* October 1 (2004), 1538.

[3] Zuberbier, T., G. Edenharter, M. Worm, I. Ehlers, S. Reimann, T. Hantke, C. C. Roehr, K. E. Bergmann, and B. Niggemann. "Prevalence of adverse reactions to food in Germany–a population study." *Allergy* 59, no. 3 (2004): 338-345.

[4] Barajas, Martín Bedolla "Frequency and Characterization of Oral Allergy Syndrome in Mexican Adults with Nasal Pollinosis," Abstracts of the XXII World Allergy Congress, 4-8 December, 2012 Cancun, Mexico. February 2012 - Volume 5 - Supplement 2, #431.

[5] Barajas (2012)

[6] See the website for the U.S. Federal Food and Drug Administration
http://www.fda.gov/ForConsumers/ByAudience/ForWomen/ucm118492.htm

[7] Maeda, Nobuko, Naoko Inomata, Akiko Morita, Mio Kirino, and Zenro Ikezawa. "Correlation of oral allergy syndrome due to plant-derived foods with pollen sensitization in Japan." *Annals of Allergy, Asthma & Immunology* 104, no. 3 (2010): 205-210.

[8] Ma, Songhui, Scott H. Sicherer, and Anna Nowak-Wegrzyn. "A survey on the management of pollen-food allergy syndrome in allergy practices." *Journal of allergy and clinical immunology* 112, no. 4 (2003): 784-788.

[9] While birch, ragweed, mugwort and grass are the most common pollens that cause OAS, one Japanese study also applies the term OAS to those who suffer from Japan cedar pollinosis, in which sufferers react to melon, apple, peach, and kiwi fruit amongst other foods. Ishida T, Murai K, Yasuda T, Satou T, Sejima T, Kitamura K., "Oral allergy syndrome in patients with Japanese cedar pollinosis," *Nihon Jibiinkoka Gakkai Kaiho,* March;103, no. 3 (2000):199-205.

[10] Skypala, I. J., S. Bull, K. Deegan, K. Gruffydd-Jones, S. Holmes, I. Small, P. W. Emery, and S. R. Durham. "The prevalence of pollen-food syndrome (PFS) and prevalence and characteristics of reported food allergy; a survey of UK adults aged 18-75 incorporating a validated PFS diagnostic questionnaire." *Clinical & Experimental Allergy* (2013).

[11] General information on oral allergy syndrome, such as symptoms and food associated with it, has been compiled based on the numerous sources cited in this reference section.

[12] This chart was compiled based on a wide variety of research and from foods mentioned in relation to oral allergy syndrome in the various studies cited throughout this book. The basis of this chart comes from the Canadian Food Inspection Agency's website, and information from the Calgary Allergy Network. Information on latex comes from Wagner, S. and Breiteneder, H. "The latex-fruit syndrome", *Biochemical Society transaction,* November 2002, 30 (Pt 6): 935-940. Dates are not often included on OAS charts, but have been found to cross react with both birch and timothy grass, see A. A. A. Kwaasi1, H. A. Harfi, R. S. Parhar, S. Saleh, K. S. Collison, R. C. Panzani, S. T. Al-Sedairy, F. A. Al-Mohanna1, "Cross-reactivities between date palm (Phoenix dactylifera L.) polypeptides and foods implicated in the oral allergy syndrome," *Allergy,* Volume 57, Issue 6, pages 508–518, June (2002).

[13] Cypress has fairly recently been associated with oral allergy syndrome. This appears to be a more common problem in Japan, where many people have recently been diagnosed with oral allergy syndrome, as well as allergies to Japanese Cedar, a subspecies of cypress. See Sánchez-López, J., et al. "Cupressus arizonica Pollen: A New Pollen Involved in the Lipid Transfer Protein Syndrome?," *Journal of Investigational Allergology and Clinical Immunology* 21.7 (2011): 522; M. San Miguel-Moncín,*et al.* "Lettuce anaphylaxis: identification of a lipid transfer protein as the major allergen," *Allergy,* Volume 58, Issue 6, pages 511–517, June 2003; Maeda (2010); Morita A, Kondou M, Shirai T, Ikezawa Z., "Occupational Contact Urticaria Syndrome Caused By Handling Lettuce and Chicory: Cross-reactivity Between Lettuce and Chicory," *Journal of Allergy and Clinical Immunology,* 2007;119:S24.

[14] Westman, Marit, Anna Asarnoj, Inger Kull, Marianne van Hage, Magnus Wickman, and Elina Toskala, "Natural course and comorbidities of allergic and nonallergic rhinitis in children," *Journal of Allergy and Clinical Immunology,* Volume 129, Issue 2, February 2012, page 407.

[15] Saarinen K, Jantunen J, Haahtela T, "Birch Pollen Honey for Birch Pollen Allergy – A Randomized Controlled Pilot Study," *International Archives of Allergy and Immunology,* 155:160-166 (2011), 162.

[16] Gretchen Cuda Kroen, "Ticked Off About a Growing Allergy to Meat," *Sciencemag.org,* 16 November 2012 http://news.sciencemag.org/sciencenow/2012/11/ticked-off-about-a-growing-aller.html?ref=hp

[17] Okamoto Y, Kurihara K., "A case of oral allergy syndrome whose symptoms were dramatically improved after rush subcutaneous injection immunotherapy with pollen extracts of birch," *Arerugi* 2012 May;61(5):652-8.

[18] Mauro, Marina, Marina Russello, Cristoforo Incorvaia, Gianbattista Gazzola, Franco Frati, Philippe Moingeon, Gianni Passalacqua, "Birch-Apple Syndrome Treated with Birch Pollen Immunotherapy," *International Archives of Allergy and Immunotherapy,* Vol. 156, No. 4 (2011).

[19] K. Saarinen (2011)

[20] Warner JO, Kaliner MA, Crisci CD, et al. "Allergy practice worldwide – A report by the World Allergy Organization Specialty and Training Counsel." *Allergy & Clinical Immunology International - Journal of the World Allergy Organization* 2006;18:4-10

[21] Kellberger, Jessica, Holger Dressel, Christian Vogelberg, Wolfgang Leupold, Doris Windstetter, Gudrun Weinmayr, Jon Genuneit et al. "Prediction of the incidence and persistence of allergic rhinitis in adolescence: a prospective cohort study." Journal of Allergy and Clinical Immunology 129, no. 2 (2012): 397-402; Kim, Woo

Kyung, Ji-Won Kwon, Ju-Hee Seo, Hyung Young Kim, Jinho Yu, Byoung-Ju Kim, Hyo-Bin Kim et al. "Interaction between< i> IL13</i> genotype and environmental factors in the risk for allergic rhinitis in Korean children," *Journal of Allergy and Clinical Immunology* 130, no. 2 (2012): 421-426.

[22] Wang, De-Yun. "Risk factors of allergic rhinitis: genetic or environmental?," *Therapeutics and clinical risk management* 1, no. 2 (2005): 115.

[23] Räsänen, M., T. Laitinen, J. Kaprio, M. Koskenvuo, and L. A. Laitinen. "Hay fever—a Finnish nationwide study of adolescent twins and their parents." *Allergy* 53, no. 9 (1998): 885-890; Schultz Larsen, Finn, Niels V. Holm, and Klavs Henningsen. "Atopic dermatitis: a genetic-epidemiologic study in a population-based twin sample." *Journal of the American Academy of Dermatology* 15, no. 3 (1986): 487-494.

[24] Maeda, (2010).

[25] Skypala, (2013).

[26] Kondrashova, Anita, Tapio Seiskari, Jorma Ilonen, Mikael Knip, and Heikki Hyöty. "The 'Hygiene hypothesis' and the sharp gradient in the incidence of autoimmune and allergic diseases between Russian Karelia and Finland." *Apmis* (2012), 479.

[27] Illi, Sabina, Erika von Mutius, Susanne Lau, Renate Bergmann, Bodo Niggemann, Christine Sommerfeld, and Ulrich Wahn. "Early childhood infectious diseases and the development of asthma up to school age: a birth cohort study." *Bmj* 322, no. 7283 (2001): 390-395; Kondrashova, (2012)

[28] "Dodging antibiotic side effects." Wyss Institute at Harvard University, Date: Jul 3, 2013 http://wyss.harvard.edu/viewpressrelease/117/ ; M. Mai1, I. Kull, M. Wickman, A. Bergström, "Antibiotic use in early life and development of allergic diseases: respiratory infection as the explanation," *Clinical & Experimental Allergy*, Volume 40 Issue 8, August (2010).

[29] See note 28.

[30] M. Mai1 (2010)

[31] Guarner, Francisco, and Juan-R. Malagelada. "Gut flora in health and disease," *The Lancet,* 361, no. 9356 (2003): 512-519.

[32] Bisgaard, Hans, Nan Li, Klaus Bonnelykke, Bo Lund Krogsgaard Chawes, Thomas Skov, Georg Paludan-Müller, Jakob Stokholm, Birgitte Smith, and Karen Angeliki Krogfelt. "Reduced diversity of the intestinal microbiota during infancy is associated with increased risk of allergic disease at school age," *Journal of Allergy and Clinical Immunology,* 128, no. 3 (2011): 646-652; Kukkonen, Kaarina, Mikael Kuitunen, Tari Haahtela, Riitta Korpela, Tuija Poussa, and Erkki Savilahti. "High intestinal IgA associates with reduced risk of IgE-associated allergic diseases," *Pediatric Allergy and Immunology* 21, no. 1-Part-I (2010): 67-73.

[33] Penders, John, Carel Thijs, Cornelis Vink, Foekje F. Stelma, Bianca Snijders, Ischa Kummeling, Piet A. van den Brandt, and Ellen E. Stobberingh. "Factors influencing the composition of the intestinal microbiota in early infancy." *Pediatrics* 118, no. 2 (2006): 511-521.

[34] Forsythe, Paul, Mark D. Inman, and John Bienenstock. "Oral treatment with live Lactobacillus reuteri inhibits the allergic airway response in mice." *American journal of respiratory and critical care medicine* 175, no. 6 (2007): 561-569; Kukkonen, (2010); Singh, A., F. Hacini-Rachinel, M. L. Gosoniu, T. Bourdeau, S. Holvoet, R. Doucet-Ladeveze, M. Beaumont, A. Mercenier, and S. Nutten. "Immune-modulatory effect of probiotic Bifidobacterium lactis NCC2818 in individuals suffering from seasonal allergic rhinitis to grass pollen: an exploratory, randomized, placebo-controlled clinical trial." *European journal of clinical nutrition* 67, no. 2 (2013): 161-167; Wang, Ming Fuu,

Hsiao Chuan Lin, Ying Yu Wang, and Ching Hsiang Hsu. "Treatment of perennial allergic rhinitis with lactic acid bacteria." *Pediatric allergy and immunology* 15, no. 2 (2004): 152-158; Wassenberg, J., S. Nutten, R. Audran, N. Barbier, V. Aubert, J. Moulin, A. Mercenier, and F. Spertini. "Effect of Lactobacillus paracasei ST11 on a nasal provocation test with grass pollen in allergic rhinitis." *Clinical & Experimental Allergy* 41, no. 4 (2011): 565-573; Yonekura, Syuji, Yoshitaka Okamoto, Toru Okawa, Minako Hisamitsu, Hideaki Chazono, Kouichi Kobayashi, Daiju Sakurai, Shigetoshi Horiguchi, and Toyoyuki Hanazawa. "Effects of daily intake of Lactobacillus paracasei strain KW3110 on Japanese cedar pollinosis." In *Allergy and Asthma Proceedings*, vol. 30, no. 4, pp. 397-405. OceanSide Publications, Inc, 2009.

[35] Maslova, Ekaterina, Thorhallur I. Halldorsson, Marin Strøm, and Sjurdur F. Olsen. "Low-fat yoghurt intake in pregnancy associated with increased child asthma and allergic rhinitis risk: a prospective cohort study." *Journal of Nutritional Science* 1 (2012).

[36] Yonekura, (2009)

[37] Penders, John, Carel Thijs, Cornelis Vink, Foekje F. Stelma, Bianca Snijders, Ischa Kummeling, Piet A. van den Brandt, and Ellen E. Stobberingh. "Factors influencing the composition of the intestinal microbiota in early infancy." *Pediatrics* 118, no. 2 (2006): 511-521, 512.

[38] Penders, (2006), 516-517.

[39] Pender, 520.

[40] Lu, Chan, QiHong Deng, CuiYun Ou, WeiWei Liu, and Jan Sundell. "Effects of ambient air pollution on allergic rhinitis among preschool children in Changsha, China," *Chinese Science Bulletin* (2013): 1-7, 3.

[41] Seo, Ju-Hee, Hyung Young Kim, Young-Ho Jung, Ji-Won Kwon, Byoung-Ju Kim, Hyo-Bin Kim, Woo Kyung Kim et al. "The association between sibling and allergic rhinitis in adolescents," *Allergy Asthma & Respiratory Disease* 1, no. 1 (2013): 67-72.

[42] Penders, John, Kerstin Gerhold, Ellen E. Stobberingh, Carel Thijs, Kurt Zimmermann, Susanne Lau, and Eckard Hamelmann. "Establishment of the intestinal microbiota and its role for atopic dermatitis in early childhood," *Journal of Allergy and Clinical Immunology* (2013).

[43] Muehleisen, Beda, and Richard L. Gallo. "Vitamin D in allergic disease: Shedding light on a complex problem." *Journal of Allergy and Clinical Immunology* 131, no. 2 (2013): 324-329, 326. Citing this study: Vahavihu K, Ala-Houhala M, Peric M, Karisola P, Kautiainen H, Hasan T, et al. "Narrowband ultraviolet B treatment improves vitamin D balance and alters antimicrobial peptide expression in skin lesions of psoriasis and atopic dermatitis," *British Journal of Dermatology,* 2010;163:321-8.

[44] Muehleisen, 326 citing: Sharief S, Jariwala S, Kumar J, Muntner P, Melamed ML. Vitamin D levels and food and environmental allergies in the United States: results from the National Health and Nutrition Examination Survey 2005-2006. *Journal of Allergy and Clinical Immunology,* 2011;127:1195-202

[45] Jones, Mitchell L., Christopher J. Martoni, and Satya Prakash. "Oral supplementation with probiotic L. reuteri NCIMB 30242 increases mean circulating 25-hydroxyvitamin D: a post-hoc analysis of a randomized controlled trial," *Journal of Clinical Endocrinology & Metabolism* (2013).

[46] Bartle, Janette, and Jean Emberlin. "Understanding the main causes of hayfever," *Practice Nursing* 22, no. 5, 2011: 231-235; Stöcklin, Laura, Georg Loss, Erika von Mutius, Jon Genuneit, Elisabeth Horak, and Charlotte Braun-Fahrländer. "Health-related quality of life does not explain the protective effect of farming on allergies," *Pediatric Allergy and Immunology* 23, no. 6 (2012): 519-521, 520; Wlasiuk, Gabriela, and Donata Vercelli. "The farm effect, or: when, what and how a farming environment protects from asthma and allergic disease," *Current Opinion in*

Allergy and Clinical Immunology 12, no. 5 (2012): 461-466. This article provides an overview of research on the protective effects of farming as well as the three main factors associated with asthma and AR – exposure to a wide diversity of microbes, maternal ingestion of unprocessed milk, and exposure to farm animals; Ziska, Lewis H., and Paul J. Beggs. "Anthropogenic climate change and allergen exposure: the role of plant biology." *Journal of Allergy and Clinical Immunology* 129, no. 1 (2012): 27-32.

[47] Wlasiuk, (2012)

[48] Wlasiuk, (2012)

[49] Lampi, J., D. Canoy, D. Jarvis, A-L. Hartikainen, L. Keski-Nisula, M-R. Järvelin, and J. Pekkanen. "Farming environment and prevalence of atopy at age 31: prospective birth cohort study in Finland," *Clinical & Experimental Allergy,* 41, no. 7 (2011): 987-993.

[50] Eriksson, J., L. Ekerljung, J. Lötvall, T. Pullerits, G. Wennergren, Eva Rönmark, K. Toren, and B. Lundbäck. "Growing up on a farm leads to lifelong protection against allergic rhinitis," *Allergy* 65, no. 11 (2010): 1397-1403.

[51] Ziska, (2012)

[52] Ziska, (2012)

[53] Hodgekiss, Anna. "Hay fever playing up? Blame the birch trees and steer clear of celery!" *dailymail.co.uk* March 19, 2012. http://www.dailymail.co.uk/health/article-2117342/Hay-fever-playing-Blame-birch-trees-steer-clear-celery.html#ixzz2SkdwD77P

[54] Lu, Chan (2013); Altuğ, Hicran, Eftade O. Gaga, Tuncay Döğeroğlu, Özlem Özden, Sermin Örnektekin, Bert Brunekreef, Kees Meliefste, Gerard Hoek, and Wim Van Doorn. "Effects of air pollution on lung function and symptoms of asthma, rhinitis and eczema in primary school children," *Environmental Science and Pollution Research* (2013): 1-13.

[55] Smith, Laurence C., *The World in 2050: Four Forces Shaping Civilization's Northern Future,* New York: Dutton, 2010, 129.

Englander, John., *High Tide on Main Street: Rising Sea Level and the Coming Coastal Crisis*, Boca Raton, Florida: The Science Bookshelf, 2012, 40.

[56] Ziska, (2012)

[57] Ziska, Lewis, Kim Knowlton, Christine Rogers, Dan Dalan, Nicole Tierney, Mary Ann Elder, Warren Filley et al. "Recent warming by latitude associated with increased length of ragweed pollen season in central North America." *Proceedings of the National Academy of Sciences* 108, no. 10 (2011): 4248-4251.

[58] García-Mozo, Herminia, Carmen Galán, Victoria Jato, Jordina Belmonte, Consuelo Díaz de la Guardia, Delia Fernández, Montserrat Gutiérrez et al. "Quercus pollen season dynamics in the Iberian Peninsula: response to meteorological parameters and possible consequences of climate change," *Annals of Agricultural and Environmental Medicine,* 13, no. 2 (2006): 209.

[59] Athanasios Damialis, John M. Halley, Dimitrios Gioulekas, Despina Vokou, "Long-term trends in atmospheric pollen levels in the city of Thessaloniki, Greece," *Atmospheric Environment*, Volume 41, Issue 33, October 2007, Pages 7011–7021.

[60] Stach, A., H. Garcia-Mozo, J. C. Prieto-Baena, M. Czarnecka-Operacz, D. Jenerowicz, W. Silny, and C. Galán. "Prevalence of Artemisia Species Pollinosis in Western Poland: Impact of Climate Change on Aerobiological

Trends," *Journal of Investigational Allergology and Clinical Immunology,* 17, no. 1 (2007): 39-47. http://www.jiaci.org/issues/vol17issue01/7.pdf

[61] Frei, Thomas, and Ewald Gassner. "Climate change and its impact on birch pollen quantities and the start of the pollen season an example from Switzerland for the period 1969–2006," *International Journal of Biometeorology,* 52, no. 7 (2008): 667-674.

[62] Rasmussen, Alix. "The effects of climate change on the birch pollen season in Denmark," *Aerobiologia,* 18, no. 3-4 (2002): 253-265.

[63] Athanasios, (2007), 1.

[64] García-Mozo, (2007), 1.

[65] Ziska, Lewis H., and Frances A. Caulfield. "Rising CO_2 and pollen production of common ragweed (Ambrosia artemisiifolia L.), a known allergy-inducing species: implications for public health." *Functional Plant Biology* 27, no. 10 (2000): 893-898.

[66] Hernandez, Evelia, Albino Barraza-Villarreal, Maria Consuelo Escamilla-Nunez, Leticia Hernandez-Cadena, Peter D. Sly, Lynnette Marie Neufeld, Usha Ramakishnan, and Isabelle Romieu. "Prenatal determinants of cord blood total immunoglobulin E levels in Mexican newborns," *Allergy and Asthma Proceedings*, vol. 34, no. 5, pp. e27-e34. OceanSide Publications, Inc, 2013.

[67] Jerschow, Elina, Aileen P. McGinn, Gabriele de Vos, Natalia Vernon, Sunit Jariwala, Golda Hudes, and David Rosenstreich. "Dichlorophenol-containing pesticides and allergies: results from the US National Health and Nutrition Examination Survey 2005-2006," *Annals of Allergy, Asthma & Immunology* (2012).

[68] Slager, Rebecca E., Jill A. Poole, Tricia D. LeVan, Dale P. Sandler, Michael CR Alavanja, and Jane A. Hoppin. "Rhinitis associated with pesticide exposure among commercial pesticide applicators in the Agricultural Health Study," *Occupational and environmental medicine,* 66, no. 11 (2009): 718-724.

[69] Chatzi, Leda, Athanasios Alegakis, Nikolaos Tzanakis, Nikolaos Siafakas, Manolis Kogevinas, and Christos Lionis. "Association of allergic rhinitis with pesticide use among grape farmers in Crete, Greece," *Occupational and environmental medicine,* 64, no. 6 (2007): 417-421.

[70] Bernstein, I. Leonard, Jonathan A. Bernstein, Maureen Miller, Sylva Tierzieva, David I. Bernstein, Zana Lummus, M. K. Selgrade, Donald L. Doerfler, and Verner L. Seligy. "Immune responses in farm workers after exposure to Bacillus thuringiensis pesticides," *Environmental Health Perspectives,* 107, no. 7 (1999): 575.

[71] Aris, Aziz, and Samuel Leblanc. "Maternal and fetal exposure to pesticides associated to genetically modified foods in Eastern Townships of Quebec, Canada," *Reproductive Toxicology* 31, no. 4 (2011): 528-533.

[72] Mendell, Mark J. "Indoor residential chemical emissions as risk factors for respiratory and allergic effects in children: a review," *Indoor air* 17, no. 4 (2007): 259-277. This particular paper is an assessment of 21 studies on the effects of indoor air pollutants on allergies and asthma.

Nurmatov, U., Nara Tagieva, Sean Semple, Graham Devereux, and Aziz Sheikh. "Volatile organic compounds and risk of asthma and allergy: a systematic review and meta-analysis of observational and interventional studies," *Primary care respiratory journal: journal of the General Practice Airways Group* 22, no. 1 (2013): PS9-PS15. This particular paper is an assessment of the recent studies on the effects of volatile organic compounds in preparation for further research.

[73] Kim, Haejin, and Jonathan A. Bernstein. "Air pollution and allergic disease," *Current allergy and asthma reports,* 9, no. 2 (2009): 128-133.

[74] Diaz-Sanchez, David, Robert Rumold, and Henry Gong Jr. "Challenge with environmental tobacco smoke exacerbates allergic airway disease in human beings," *Journal of allergy and clinical immunology,* 118, no. 2 (2006): 441-446.

[75] Schnuch, A., E. Oppel, T. Oppel, H. Römmelt, M. Kramer, E. Riu, U. Darsow, B. Przybilla, D. Nowak, and R. A. Jörres. "Experimental inhalation of fragrance allergens in predisposed subjects: effects on skin and airways," *British Journal of Dermatology,* 162, no. 3 (2010): 598-606.

[76] Hsu, Nai-Yun, et al. "Feeding bottles usage and the prevalence of childhood allergy and asthma," *Clinical and Developmental Immunology,* (2012); Midoro-Horiuti, Terumi, Ruby Tiwari, Cheryl S. Watson, and Randall M. Goldblum. "Maternal bisphenol a exposure promotes the development of experimental asthma in mouse pups," *Environmental health perspectives,* 118, no. 2 (2010): 273.

[77] For the European Union, see http://www.efsa.europa.eu/en/topics/topic/bisphenol.htm ; For Canada, Japan, Turkey, Denmark, and France see http://www.forbes.com/sites/michellemaisto/2012/03/05/bpa-in-food-packaging-fda-to-decide-by-march-31/

[78] Hsu, (2012)

[79] Magnusson, Jessica, Inger Kull, Helen Rosenlund, Niclas Håkansson, Alicja Wolk, Erik Melén, Magnus Wickman, and Anna Bergström. "Fish consumption in infancy and development of allergic disease up to age 12 y," *The American journal of clinical nutrition,* 97, no. 6 (2013): 1324-1330.

[80] Nwaru BI, Erkkola M, Ahonen S, Kaila M, Haapala AM, Kronberg-Kippilä C, et al. "Age at the introduction of solid foods during the first year and allergic sensitization at age 5 years," *Pediatrics,* 2010;125:50-9.

[81] MacLean, Emily, Norman Madsen, Harissios Vliagoftis, Catherine Field, and Lisa Cameron. "n-3 Fatty acids inhibit transcription of human IL-13: implications for development of T helper type 2 immune responses," *British Journal of Nutrition,* 1, no. 1 (2013): 1-11.

[82] Barg, Wojciech, Wojciech Medrala, and Anna Wolanczyk-Medrala. "Exercise-induced anaphylaxis: an update on diagnosis and treatment," *Current Allergy and Asthma Reports,* 11, no. 1 (2011): 45-51, 47.

[83] Wojciech, 2011, 47.

[84] Wojciech, 2011, 46.

[85] Wojciech, 2011, 46.

[86] Wojciech, 2011, 46.

[87] *National Institute of Allergy and Infectious Diseases,* http://www.niaid.nih.gov/topics/foodallergy/understanding/Pages/OASExercise-inducedFA.aspx

[88] Hiragun M, et al., "The sensitivity and clinical course of patients with wheat-dependent exercise-induced anaphylaxis sensitized to hydrolyzed wheat protein in facial soap," *Arerugi.* 2011 Dec;60(12):1630-40.

[89] Wojciech, 2011, 46.

[90] Wojciech, 2011, 48; *National Institute of Allergy and Infectious Diseases,*

http://www.niaid.nih.gov/topics/foodallergy/understanding/Pages/OASExercise-inducedFA.aspx; Yin, Jia, and Li-ping Wen. "Wheat-dependant Exercise-induced Anaphylaxis Clinical and Laboratory Findings in 15 Cases." *Chinese Journal of Allergy and Clinical Immunology* 1 (2010): 008.

[91] Lieberman, Phillip, Richard A. Nicklas, John Oppenheimer, Stephen F. Kemp, David M. Lang, David I. Bernstein, Jonathan A. Bernstein et al. "The diagnosis and management of anaphylaxis practice parameter: 2010 update," *Journal of Allergy and Clinical Immunology,* 126, no. 3 (2010): 477-480, 479.

[92] Tanaka, Aya, Saori Itoi, Mika Terao, Saki Matsui, Mamori Tani, Takaaki Hanafusa, Ken Igawa et al. "Food Allergy Case Reports: 424 Wheat-dependent Exercise-induced Anaphylaxis Occurred in OAS Patient after Using Soap Containing Hydrolyzed Wheat Proteins: Effect of Soap on Keratinocyte Inflammasome," *The World Allergy Organization Journal* 5, no. Suppl 2 (2012): S152.

[93] Tanaka, (2012)

[94] Hiragun M, (2011)

[95] Guillet, G., and M. H. Guillet. "Percutaneous sensitization to almond oil in infancy and study of ointments in 27 children with food allergy," *Allergie et immunologie,* 32, no. 8 (2000): 309; Kanny, G., C. Hauteclocque, and D. A. Moneret-Vautrin. "Sesame seed and sesame seed oil contain masked allergens of growing importance," *Allergy* 51, no. 12 (1996): 952-957; Maddocks-Jennings, W. "Critical incident: idiosyncratic allergic reactions to essential oils," *Complementary Therapies in Nursing and Midwifery,* 10, no. 1 (2004): 58-60.

[96] Alessandro Fiocchi, Patrizia Restani, Luca Bernardo, Alberto Martelli, Cinzia Ballabio, Enza D'Auria and Enrica Riva, "Tolerance of heat-treated kiwi by children with kiwifruit allergy," *Pediatric Allergy and Immunology,* 2004 Oct;15(5):454-8. See also Jennifer S. Kim and Scott Sicherer, "Should avoidance of foods be strict in prevention and treatment of food allergy?" *Current Opinion in Allergy and Clinical Immunology,* 2010, 10:252–257

[97] M. Fernandez-Rivas, and M. Cuevas. "Peels of Rosaceae fruits have a higher allergenicity than pulps," *Clinical and Experimental Allergy,* 29 (1999): 1239-1247; Brenna, Oreste, Carlo Pompei, Claudio Ortolani, Valerio Pravettoni, Elide A. Pastorello, and Laura Farioli, "Technological processes to decrease the allergenicity of peach juice and nectar," *Journal of Agricultural and Food Chemistry,* 48, no. 2 (2000): 493-497; Varjonen, E., E. Vainio, K. Kalimo, and K. Juntunen-Backman. "Clinical importance of non-specific lipid transfer proteins as food allergens," *Biochemical Society Transactions* 30, no. part 6 (2002), pg 3; Brenna, Oreste V., Elide A. Pastorello, Laura Farioli, Valerio Pravettoni, and Carlo Pompei. "Presence of allergenic proteins in different peach (Prunus persica) cultivars and dependence of their content on fruit ripening," *Journal of agricultural and food chemistry,* 52, no. 26 (2004): 7997-8000.

[98] Brenna, (2004); Mills, E. N., Ana I. Sancho, Neil M. Rigby, John A. Jenkins, and Alan R. Mackie. "Impact of food processing on the structural and allergenic properties of food allergens," *Molecular Nutrition & Food Research,* 53, no. 8 (2009): 963-969; Varjonen, E., E. Vainio, K. Kalimo, and K. Juntunen-Backman. "Clinical importance of non-specific lipid transfer proteins as food allergens," *Biochemical Society Transactions,* 30, no. part 6 (2002), pg 3.

[99] Jankiewicz, A., H. Aulepp, W. Baltes, K. W. Bögl, L. I. Dehne, T. Zuberbier, and S. Vieths. "Allergic sensitization to native and heated celery root in pollen-sensitive patients investigated by skin test and IgE binding." *International archives of allergy and immunology* 111, no. 3 (1996): 268-278.

[100] Nowak-Węgrzyn, Anna, Amal H. Assa'ad, Sami L. Bahna, S. Allan Bock, Scott H. Sicherer, and Suzanne S. Teuber. "Work Group report: oral food challenge testing," *Journal of Allergy and Clinical Immunology,* 123, no. 6 (2009): S365-S383.

[101] Midoro-Horiuti, (2010), and Bienkowski, Brian and Environmental Health News, "New Study Links BPA and Childhood Asthma," *Scientific American,* March 1, 2013.

[102] Anna Sapone, Julio C Bai, Carolina Ciacci, Jernej Dolinsek, Peter HR Green, Marios Hadjivassiliou, Katri Kaukinen, Kamran Rostami, David S Sanders, Michael Schumann, Reiner Ullrich, Danilo Villalta, Umberto Volta, Carlo Catassi1, and Alessio Fasano, "Spectrum of gluten-related disorders: consensus on new nomenclature and classification," *BMC Medicine* 2012, available online at: http://www.biomedcentral.com/1741-7015/10/13

[103] Walusiak J, Hanke W, Górski P, Pałczyński C, "Respiratory allergy in apprentice bakers: do occupational allergies follow the allergic march?" *Allergy* 2004, **59**:442-450

[104] Franck, P., G. Kanny, B. Dousset, P. Nabet, and D. A. Moneret-Vautrin. "Lettuce allergy." *Allergy* 55, no. 2 (2000): 201-202; Krook, Gösta. "Simultaneous occurrence of immediate and delayed allergy as a cause of contact dermatitis," *Contact Dermatitis,* 3, no. 1 (1977): 27-36; Miguel-Moncín, San, M. Krail, S. Scheurer, E. Enrique, R. Alonso, A. Conti, A. Cisteró-Bahíma, and S. Vieths. "Lettuce anaphylaxis: identification of a lipid transfer protein as the major allergen," *Allergy,* 58, no. 6 (2003): 511-517; Morita, A., N. Inomata, M. Kondou, T. Shirai, and Z. Ikezawa. "Occupational Contact Urticaria Syndrome Caused By Handling Lettuce And Chicory: Cross-reactivity Between Lettuce And Chicory," *Journal of Allergy and Clinical Immunology,* 119, no. 1 (2007): S24.

[105] Pastorello, Elide Anna, Joseph Scibilia, Laura Farioli, L. Primavesi, M. G. Giuffrida, A. Mascheri, M. Piantanida et al. "Rice Allergy Demonstrated by Double-Blind Placebo-Controlled Food Challenge in Peach-Allergic Patients Is Related to Lipid Transfer Protein Reactivity," *International archives of allergy and immunology,* 161, no. 3 (2013): 265-273.

[106] Villalta, D., G. Longo, and G. Mistrello. "A case of rice allergy in a patient with baker's asthma." *European annals of allergy and clinical immunology* 44, no. 5 (2012): 207-209.

[107] Trcka, Jiri, Susanne G. Schäd, Stephan Scheurer, Amedeo Conti, Stefan Vieths, Gerd Gross, and Axel Trautmann. "Rice-induced anaphylaxis: IgE-mediated allergy against a 56-kDa glycoprotein," *International archives of allergy and immunology,* 158, no. 1 (2011): 9-17.

[108] "Watermelon May Have Viagra-Effect," *ScienceDaily.com*, July 1, 2008 http://www.sciencedaily.com/releases/2008/06/080630165707.htm

INDEX

Made in the USA
Monee, IL
28 April 2021

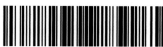